CANCER
is my teacher

LUCY O'DONNELL

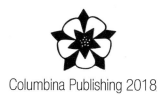

Columbina Publishing 2018

First published in 2014 by Quartet Books Limited
Reprinted (twice) 2014
This edition 2018
Published by Columbina Publishing
Copyright © Lucy O'Donnell 2014
The right of Lucy O'Donnell to be identified
as the author of this work has been asserted
by her in accordance with the
Copyright, Designs and Patents Act, 1988
A catalogue record for this book
is available from the British Library
ISBN 9781717876928
Typeset by Josh Bryson
Printed and bound using
Amazon Kindle Direct Publishing

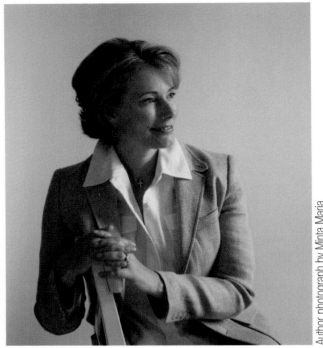

Lucy O'Donnell's passion for healthy living propelled her to start her multi-award-winning granola cereal business, Lovedean Granola. She is a former 'Entrepreneur of the Year' and a nominee for 'Woman of the Year'.

When Lucy was diagnosed with Stage 4 metastatic breast cancer in November 2011, she spent most of the next eighteen months in radical cancer treatment.

Through this continuing experience Lucy has channelled her energies into helping other people in the cancer world, and she is now both an author and a cancer life coach.

Lucy lives in West Sussex with her husband and three children.

Every two minutes someone in the UK is diagnosed with cancer. Lucy O'Donnell was one herself three years ago. Cancer is My Teacher is her story, describing unflinchingly how she has turned the disease into a positive experience – and how other people can do the same.

Lucy's approach is determined but disciplined, clinical but also holistic. By addressing the physical, emotional, and spiritual aspects of cancer, Lucy covers the whole spectrum of the disease – including how to tell the family, the dos and don'ts of communicating with apatient, the side-effects of radiotherapy and chemotherapy – and gives practical advice on how to keep looking your best and even what to pack for surgery.

Cancer is My Teacher offers guidance for anyone in the early stages of diagnosis, in treatment or trying to readjust afterwards. It also helps family and loved ones to understand what they're going through – and, above all, carries a message of hope for everyone touched by cancer.

Contents

To Matt Gordon and everybody else
who has left this world too early

What Cancer Cannot Do

It cannot cripple love
It cannot shatter hope
It cannot corrode faith
It cannot destroy peace
It cannot kill friendships
It cannot suppress memories
It cannot silence courage
It cannot invade the soul
It cannot steal eternal life
It cannot conquer the spirit

– Anon

Foreword

It is an honour to be asked to write the foreword to Cancer is My Teacher.

I have seen many books in the past written about cancer from a patient's perspective but rarely have I seen an account that is so extraordinarily intimate and yet remains soberly factual and full of common sense and practical advice about how to cope during the arduous journey through the cancer treatment.

While physicians like I hope to educate patients and support them with a wide group of health professionals within a multidisciplinary team we cannot know what it is like to go through the cancer journey ourselves. What this book does is provide a first-hand account full of hope and positivity through the highs and lows of the cancer journey from diagnosis to the completion of treatment. It is full of real life practical tips on how to handle many varied experiences and I know that this will be of huge help to patients not just with breast cancer but those with any form of cancer as well as those caring for them as they are going through this experience.

It is a privilege to be able to care for Lucy O'Donnell and her determination to 'live positively with her cancer and its treatment' has been an inspiration for me.

Paul Ellis MD FRACP, Professor of Medical Oncology

Preface

I have learnt so much about life, love and survival since my diagnosis of incurable breast cancer in November 2011 – and I would like to share this with you. My book is intended to be a comfort emotionally and practically, not just to those with cancer but also, just as importantly, to friends, family and colleagues.

My thanks and love goes out to everybody who has been, and still is, with me on my journey.

With light and love,
Lucy
September, 2014

On 3rd November 2011, when I was 46 years old, I was diagnosed with 'Stage 4 Advanced Breast Cancer' that had metastasised (spread) to my bone and liver. On the very day after my diagnosis I started a journal. There were many reasons for this. The primary being that in case I didn't make it, I would have been able to impart to my children, husband and close family how much I love them – and they would have something to keep with them and remember me by, knowing that I was still there with them in spirit. Hopefully it wouldn't come to that and the book would end up in the back of a dusty old bookshelf, long forgotten about, but I had the urge to write it anyway.

At the time I thought the journal was mainly for my family and friends, but I stopped writing it after ten days anyway. I found it extremely difficult to focus as I was more concerned with my treatment and just getting through those first few weeks, assimilating all the bucket loads of information and protocols, trying to understand what was actually happening to me and at the same time attempting to live a 'normal' life with the children. Christmas was around the corner and come hell or high water, even though I had started chemo, I was going to send out my huge pile of cards with their special Christmas message: '"If I only have one thing to say in this world, it is thank you" – Meister Eckhart.'

I was determined that nothing was going to change for my children, and to an extent, as little as possible, for my husband.

A year later, I re-read the short journal and I thought, I really must put this down on paper, a sort of 'how to' on cancer. Being diagnosed with cancer is like being struck by lightning. Apart from being a mammoth unexpected shock, the pace at which you have to deal with the news and make decisions in those first few days can leave your head spinning. So many questions and worries spring to your mind and you don't know the answers. Well, this book is aimed to help with those questions and provide information that you wouldn't otherwise get.

I remembered how, when I was diagnosed, I was given so many books that my head was literally swimming. These books were often hundreds of pages long and written in very medical terms. My book is the antithesis of this. It is supposed to be a one-stop shop, with practical, physical and emotional advice that is easy to follow and to dip into as and when needed. Once you are into chemotherapy it is often very hard to read and focus for too long. The characteristics of the particular cancer concerned will influence which chapters or sections you would want to read first, or read at all! The aim of this book will be brief, concise and to the point.

Since being diagnosed, I have been contacted by many people who have either just been diagnosed, or are living with cancer. These people want to know how I dealt with my situation. What did I do to make it easier? They have heard that I have been doing many things, coping well, and that I have adapted my lifestyle to embrace dealing with this disease with spectacular results – and they want to know what I did. So this is why I have written this book.

I hope that it will help anybody else who has just been diagnosed, or just as importantly people who have a nagging feeling about their body but don't have the courage to be pushy and seek investigation.

Very importantly – this is not a medical book. I have no medical qualifications and I am not a nutritionist. However, I have been in the 'healthy' food industry for many years and I am passionate about the subject. Also worth noting is that some of the detail is specifically about breast cancer, but much of what I am saying – i.e. side-effects and caring for yourself physically and emotionally – applies to anyone with any type of cancer.

If there is one thing that resonates more in my mind than anything else it is this: 'It Is What It Is.' Once I realised that, quite early on, and after some fantastic courses and meditations, I came to the conclusion that cancer really was my teacher.

CANCER IS MY TEACHER

1
My Life Before Cancer & Diagnosis

LISTEN TO YOUR BODY

On that day in November 2011, when I was diagnosed aged 46, I was living in the country with my husband, Carletto, and our three children, Columbus, Angelica and Archie, and a menagerie of animals. Several years before, I had started making a healthy homemade breakfast cereal, Lovedean Granola, full of natural and nutritious ingredients. I was fed up with my children eating sugary and nutritionally bare cereals, full of preservatives and additives – which basically means you are filing your body with cancer-inducing toxins. Breakfast is such an important meal, especially for children, as you never know what they are eating if they are out all day at school.

Within a few weeks, my friends and family were all ordering the cereal from me, and soon I had a little business. A prominent and very well-known London restaurateur and club owner used to send his driver down from London to pick it up. Having the thumbs up from this discerning gentleman made me realise that I really did have a good product. I was making it at home and it became a nonstop production. This was so unexpected, and I had no infrastructure, so I hired a couple of Czech au pairs to help me with the whole process which included admin, packing and delivery. At this point I was encouraged to enter it into the Great Tastes Awards, which are the Oscars of the food industry in the UK, and my granola won Gold! The highest accolade. Soon to follow were many other national awards. I was amazed and really chuffed. I realised that I was on to a big thing here and somehow I managed to retain the services of a manufacturer in the north of England that manufactured for huge cereal companies like Kellogg's. I was extremely small fry, but they gave me a chance, and they were wonderful people to work with.

My next mission was to get my product listed in Waitrose. I knew that without this I would be stuck. Waitrose loved it and listed it in 450 stores in England (that's about 80 per cent at that time). I had no marketing budget; it was just word of mouth and me. Everybody seemed obsessed by this product, and soon it was being stocked in countless other premium and high-end independent stores, such as Fortnum & Mason, and Selfridges, and many premium hotels. In Selfridges it was the twelfth best-selling grocery product. Was I chuffed or not?

I was effectively running this business myself, undertaking all the marketing/PR, sales, financials, stock, overseeing the manufacturing and so forth. I had decided to call it Lovedean (because I had to think of a name really quickly and this was the name of the village that I lived in at the time). I especially liked the fact it had the word 'love' in it – as essentially I am the sort of person who wants to nurture and create, and I was making this for the love of my children, to keep them eating healthy. I was on a crusade to highlight the criminal food additives and total rubbish that is mis-sold as nutritious and good for you.

At every possible moment I extolled the virtues of natural foods, whenever I could in my publicity – the *Daily Mail*, the *Telegraph*, *Woman & Home*, *The Grocer* and many more. I ended up becoming 'Entrepreneur of the Year' and a nominee for 'Woman of the Year' and without realising I had become the 'trailblazer' for granola (a cereal that didn't exist back then in the UK). I know, it is hard to believe as now the market is saturated with granola and related products.

Lovedean soon became more than a full-time job for one person. I had a husband and three small children to look after, so it goes without saying that I was definitely pushing my limits – but I was enjoying the challenge. I loved selling this product because it was real and made so many people happy. But equally, it was extremely tough. I was using every molecule of energy I had running Lovedean, trying to keep up my friend-ships and most importantly trying to be a great mum and wife. Something had to give – and yes, you've guessed it, unbeknown to me, it was my health. I was so busy and wired the whole time, I never had time to relax, have down time and, most importantly, listen to my body. I never gave myself time to rest, process happy events, to really enjoy life. Everything was one long list of things to do and accomplish. There was never time to recharge my batteries.

Recently, a friend told me that she has never forgotten what I said to her while Lovedean was still operating in its latter stages: that my success came at 'great personal expense'.

I began to feel unwell. This wasn't new. I had been feeling unwell for a while, but I couldn't work out if it was just the strains of my work and my lifestyle or if it was something more.

I am an energetic and productive person, used to working under pressure. But here I was, dream-ing about being taken away to a place where I could just sleep for three days. Although I ate incredibly healthily, I started to ruin it by having a very strong desire for chocolate and sugary things. Every time I walked through my kitchen (which was several times a day), I couldn't resist taking a spoonful of Nutella. I could get through a jar in two days. I suppose you could say I was addicted to it – it gave me a burst of energy, made me feel OK for a short while. The all-consuming need for sugar was constant. No wonder I had started to gain weight and look puffy and aged. (We later found out that this desire for sugar was my body crying out for it to feed my rapidly growing tumours – see plate.)

I had recently been told that I had extremely low levels of certain hormones (probably caused by fact that I had an ovary and fallopian removed at 21 years of age). Rather than taking HRT, I had discovered an ongoing treatment called 'Bio Identical Hormones' – a more natural form of hormone replacement therapy. I started this in July 2011. During that month my breast swelled up as one of the side-effects of the oestrogen. This was a perfectly normal reaction – so I didn't think too much about it and thought everything would settle down.

But as we sailed into August and September, I noticed that one breast was still more swollen than the other and extremely tender, and my armpit ached. Again, I wasn't too worried as it is very common to have breast tenderness. Breast tenderness does not mean you have cancer. And I was playing tennis quite a lot, so I had put it down to muscle ache. Still, I had a niggly feeling exacerbated by the fact that the bottom half of my breast had a very slightly pink and inflamed appearance and began to hurt a lot if one of my children bumped into me or jumped on me in the morning, to say hello, which Archie, my youngest, tends to do on a regular basis.

Having been to my local NHS GP on numerous occasions complaining of feeling utterly exhausted and unwell, I went back to him on 3rd October 2011 with the above symptoms and asked for him to send me off for a mammogram. He did not seem too worried about anything and I felt a little bit of a paranoid hypochondriac. So I was hesitant, and didn't actually go for the mammogram until 3rd November, a month later.

In fact, I felt so guilty about using the NHS that I chose to go privately in the end. My local GP had said that they didn't recommend mammograms for people under 50, and that there was nothing to indicate there was anything wrong with me. If I had listened to him, I wouldn't have gone and probably wouldn't be here now.

I remember arriving at the breast cancer screening centre at 4.45pm – it was nearly dark. I was greeted by a sweet nurse who took me into a room to talk to me about what was going to happen. I remember feeling incredibly guilty that I was there and was apologetic in my demeanour.

After the mammogram (ghastly things – you feel like a cow having your udders clamped!) I was taken into another room by the consultant radiologist. I was still at this point feeling guilty for wasting all these professional people's time. The radiologist was efficient but warm. She had the results up on the screen, talked me through the pictures and pointed out the abnormalities that she had picked up, which were plain to see. She looked me straight in the eye and said, 'I am worried.'

'What do you mean?' I said.

'I am very worried,' she said.

My mouth went very dry. 'Are you saying I have cancer?'

'Without a shadow of a doubt,' was her reply.

It was a surreal moment. Tears rolled down my face as I cried silently. I was determined to keep my composure and find out as much as I could. The radiologist took my hand and held it. My first thoughts were of how I was going to look after my children and my husband and how on earth I was going to tell my parents. I wasn't ready to have a life-threatening illness. I had just come through a very stressful work period in my life and had decided to step back slightly from it. I was beginning to really start enjoying life again. I had just been thinking how lucky I was to be feeling so happy, and have such a gorgeous family, despite the exhaustion. I was looking forward to every day of my new calmer, meditative life. My second thought was that I must have been a bad person in a previous life and that this was just a punishment and if I'd been better then this wouldn't have happened.

I called my husband. I told him the news wasn't good. He was at work at the time and said he would be straight with me within the hour. This was rather good timing actually, because it meant that the radiologist could now do an ultrasound for further investigation and the relevant biopsies. The nurse was now with me, helping the radiologist and still holding my hand.

During the ultrasound, the radiologist found a suspicious-looking lymph node and more suspicious-looking tissue in the top half of my breast. She took seven biopsies. A biopsy is when a needle is used to draw sample fluid and tissue from a lump which is then tested for further information about the cancer. They took six from the breast and one from my lymph node. It was really quite painful and traumatic as there was no time for an anaesthetic to work. I lay there, still silent, tears still rolling down my face, wondering whether this was real or just a nightmare that I was soon to wake up from. By the time this had all happened and everything had been cleared up, labelled and prepared to be sent to the lab, my husband arrived. It was 6.20pm. We went into a room. He hugged me and I cried. I was very keen that he got the full picture from the radiologist – it was getting late and I knew she had stayed on for us. So no more time for tears; it was important that we got as much information out of her as possible.

Carletto and I went back into the treatment room and the radiologist explained as much as she could and the probable treatments I would undergo: definitely an 'operation'; and chemo-therapy and radiotherapy. It was too early to tell how aggressive the cancer was, how long it had been there, and whether or not it had already spread to my lymph nodes. We wouldn't know any of this until the biopsy results came through. This would take five working days.

It was explained to us that the next step would be to get us into see the surgeon once we had the results. An appointment was made for me and eight days of waiting began.

When we left the clinic, I shall never forget what Carletto said to me. Once we had got in the car, he said, 'Darling, one's enough for me!' I couldn't believe he had said that – I didn't know how to react, because one part of me felt physically sick at losing my breast and having only one, and the other part of me was overcome with adoration for him.

When the results came through five days later I was told that my cancer was HER 2+ (which means hormone positive, just one of many types of breast cancer).

Then, eight days later, after the results of my CT/PET scans, we were summoned back to the hospital by my surgeon to be told another piece of devastating news. The cancer had spread to my liver and bone. I think this was the hardest piece of news to hear in this first two weeks. The cancer had spread – metastasised – and this meant I had Stage 4 Cancer which is technically incurable. He told me in no uncertain terms that I was living with cancer for the rest of my life.

I had never seen my husband break down before. We staggered to the car to compose ourselves – thank God we didn't bump into anyone. 'You married a dud,' I cried, but Carletto told me never to say that again. He had married a 100-carat flawless diamond and couldn't live without me. I never realised how much Carletto loved me until then. I couldn't believe he had said that. Never mind a 100-carat diamond, I knew I had married a true jewel.

Having been given this shocking news, we had to pull ourselves together and go and see my elected oncologist for our first visit. What a fabulous man. He had the most fantastic patient manner, charismatic and upbeat. That, to me, is so important – and I think experts and people who have recovered from cancer will agree with me.

Why am I telling you all this? Well, really, it is a lesson to be learned – to listen to your body; listen to your hunches. My body was telling me I was not well and I was so distracted with my work and trying to be a fabulous wife and mother, too, that I just did not investigate my situation thoroughly enough. I should have been an awful lot more insistent, a lot earlier.

So please, anybody reading this, you must listen to your body. It is always telling you something.

2
Early Days

I think it important to say that in this book I am not going to use the words 'victim', 'survivor' or 'fighting a battle' – these are very negative words. I am not a victim and I am not fighting. In fact, I am not surviving; I am 'thriving'. I have cancer and I am living with it. I accept it and will do my best to deal with it. I know that by not being fearful and angry I can help control my cancer. Anger is an uncontrolled, dangerous and unhealthy energy.

I decided early on to get rid of all negativity, to use my energy to be positive and help the healing process. It sounds very clichéd but happiness depends on thoughts – keep your thoughts positive and happy, and you will be positive and happy.

A NOTE ON THE INTERNET

I have mentioned this very early on because the natural reaction of anybody who has been diagnosed with cancer is to go straight on to the internet. The internet is full of total rubbish most of the time and few sites can be trusted. The only websites you should look at are proper established ones such as those of specific, well-known and reputable cancer charities and medical organisations (see Further Information).

One thing to look out for is 'reported speech'. A journalist can basically quote anything if he uses 'reported speech' – and sometimes this is really not helpful and can cause a lot of very unnecessary angst, as the conclusions people draw can be wholly inaccurate. Believe me, I have experienced this.

TELLING PEOPLE

1. PARENTS

We decided not to tell my parents on the night I found out that I had cancer. I knew they would be devastated and I was still in shock. I didn't want them to have a sleepless night. I would wait until the morning, when I could be calm and collected, and when they could have the day to digest it all.

When I woke up rather early, having found it terribly difficult to get to sleep, Carletto was hugging me quite hard and I realised how lucky I was to have such a marvelous husband to support me. It made me laugh because he offered to make me a cup of tea. This was quite a significant step – he has only done this once before in our years of marriage, and it was undrinkable then. He is half-Italian – coffee is his thing. He doesn't 'do' or 'get' tea. I declined the offer, knowing that it would be frightful and told him that I would give him a tea lesson in the next few days so that he would be able to bring me endless cuppas over the coming months.

I was dreading the phone calls I had to make to my parents. I so wanted to be clear and calm and concise. I sat at my desk and practised over and over again what I would say: 'Hello, I have breast cancer'; 'Hello, how are you? I need to tell you something important. I have breast cancer'; 'Hello, are you sitting down...?' – and so it went on. I thought if I spoke calmly and with a flattish voice then I would stay in control. It was the word 'cancer' that threw me. I just couldn't say it without falling apart. No matter how hard I tried, I just couldn't

Here goes – deep breath. I ring them both. I can't say the word 'cancer'. I can't breathe and I finally stutter and cough it out. Mum cries, so I cry. I feel and hear the deep pain and anguish in her voice. I try to cheer her up and joke that one of us has to get it and that it's better I get it out of her four children as I have the better support system. I will be using the word 'support system' a lot, I think, as even now, at this early stage, I realise how important this is.

When I ring my father, my stepmother answers. 'Have you got a cold,' she says. 'Your voice sounds funny.' I don't know what to say, I am trying to keep it together. I tell her I do have a little cold and could she pass me on to Dad. I am trying to sound nonchalant because, if I don't, I will crack. Dad comes to the phone. 'Hello darling, do you have a cold? Julie's right – you sound rather stuffed up and muffled.' They don't know that this is my serious voice, my voice that is trying to stop me from crying. I tell him I am fine and that I have some important and serious news. Again, I cough it out. The phone is on speaker at their end. They always have their conversations on speaker as they both like to be in on the conversation together. It's very sweet.

Dad went silent and Julie did the talking. I knew that Dad was trying to take it in. I felt so dreadful for them both. After a few minutes he managed to come back to the phone and I tried to explain to him the situation as it stood.

Telling my parents was perhaps the hardest thing I have ever had to do. There is something terrible about thinking that your child may die before you.

There is no perfect way to tell people, though. You just have to do it when you think it is right and in a way that you think is right.

2. CHILDREN

With my children it was also extremely hard. The news had to remain a secret at first because my eldest, Columbus, was doing his mock Common Entrance exams two weeks later. The exams were seriously important and would determine which school he went to.

We decided to tell them in three weeks' time, which was torturous, pretending that everything was normal. After the exam. I didn't think I would tell them the whole story but I suspected that Columbus would become a cancer expert within days – just like his father.

Actually, I knew that they were less informed about cancer than my peers, so it was very important to me that when I told them, in the same breath, I assured them that Mummy was going to be OK. I shall never forget their little faces when I told them, and the way that all three reacted – each differently, I might add. The most gutting thing was when Archie, then nine, put his hand up as if in a classroom and with a very sensible and reasonable voice said, 'Are you going to die?' He asked the question that the other two were burning to ask too. My stomach lurched and I told him that I was not going to die. I told them Mummy would have to get very sick in order to get better; that the treatments were very effective but they were horrible. I told them I would lose my hair. Once they realised that it was OK, that I might look quite groovy in a wig and, later, when they saw other people's positive reactions to my appearance, they began to feel a bit better.

3. OTHERS

The only non-family person I told straightaway was Diana, a good friend of mine who lived nearby, who had come through a very aggressive cancer recently.

The painfully slow week we waited for the biopsy results was to be my research and decision week. I wanted to find out as much from her as I possibly could. Carletto and I still hadn't decided where to carry out my treatment, and we knew we had only a few days to make the decision.

Again, I choked out the 'cancer' word to Diana. I really looked forward to saying 'I have cancer' without choking or crying. I was hoping it would come soon.

Actually, it took several weeks before I could say it without having to really control my emotions.

4. SCHOOL AND OTHER PARENTS

I told each of my children's schools quite quickly. I thought it important that all the relevant teachers knew so that they could give the support to my children if needed. I made an appointment to see the heads and the form teachers. I am so glad I did this, at it meant it was out in the open, that it was acknowledged, that people would feel comfortable about asking how I was. I was trying to minimise the discomfort that people who don't know you very well feel when they are not sure whether they should mention something or not. Acknowledgement is very, very important – I have a whole section on this later in the book.

The same went for the parents of my children's contemporaries. They all found out pretty quickly and it still gives me goosebumps when I think about how they rallied round, helped, loved, and supported.

One memory of this time sticks out. It was Angelica's school fireworks night, a couple of days after diagnosis. I didn't want to go but I had to – I didn't want her to know anything was up. Carletto couldn't face it and anyway he had too much to do. He holed himself up in his office. He wanted to get my reports and data to my family GP in London so that they could be looked at over the weekend to help in the decision-making process.

On the evening in question I met darling Angelica at school at 6.15pm – she was so excited and ran off with her friends to the massive bonfire. I had a mulled wine and met up with Diana. I was so glad I had told her as she had so much information to give me. We hid in the damp bushes all evening, getting strange looks from other parents, with fireworks going over our heads, drinking weak mulled wine while we talked about it all – the options, the side-effects, the children. I learnt a lot that night. It was rather a surreal situation watching those fireworks go off, watching excited children and parents flying by and hiding in a bush talking about cancer.

Diana and her husband James came over soon after so that they could fill us in with as much information as they could, from drawing from their own experience. I also wanted Carletto to chat with him. I was very conscious that there would be no one looking out for Carletto and I thought it would be good for him to talk to another husband who had been through it in the sense of the spousal support.

HOW DO YOU TELL PEOPLE YOU DON'T KNOW WELL – OR DO YOU?

Again, there is no easy way to do this. In most cases it is not necessary to tell them, but sometimes you have to. Maybe because you start to feel faint and need to sit down while out shopping, or maybe you can't lift something. It is normally for practical reasons and for when you may need a stranger to help you with something. I found it much better to let them know I had cancer and was in the middle of chemo or whatever it was at the time, as then they would be much more receptive to helping me. Otherwise you may get funny attitudes and looks, which can be very upsetting at the time.

LOOKING AFTER YOUR PARTNER

I was very adamant that my husband had a free rein. I didn't want him using up all his energies hovering over me. It was bad enough for him as it was. I wanted him to go out and have fun, release his stress.

During my intense treatment, he went away a couple of times with the children on pre-planned holidays with friends, and I am really glad they did. I think it is really important that partners don't get sucked into the 'cancer environment' all of the time.

3
Coping

That which doesn't kill us only makes us stronger

— Nietzsche

Many people ask me how I cope. I will try to give an answer. My friendships and family are truly uplifting. I have never had such a heart full of joy and peace as I have now. I know that may sound strange, but it is true. I have got off that hamster wheel and I am now truly *living* my life. I may be living with cancer, but I am also living my life.

Since diagnosis, I actually feel healthier. My skin and eyes are clearer and, although I would say I am more fragile, I have so much more energy and joie de vivre. I am so happy to be alive and thank God for every day he gives me of this precious life.

During my first year with cancer there was very little time to think about it. There was so much to do. I wasn't able to think of the future – it took all my time, energy and emotion just to get through the treatments, endless specialist appointments, dealing with everyday life, and recovering from my weekly toxic chemo sessions, trying to keep myself in shape – I was rigorous about exercising – even if it meant just 20 minutes very slow walks with my dogs, or five or ten minutes of yoga or stretching. I set myself targets of doing some form of exercise every day. I focused on the 'now' – the present. That taught me a lot. That is what I try to do; live in the present. I know the facts and statistics about my particular cancer - they are pretty shocking – but what is the point of thinking about that? There is no time to do that if I want to enjoy my life. That's not to say that I don't have dark moments – of course I do – but most of the time I just file away these facts. I 'park' them, just like I have parked so many other things in my life now. I am glad I know them – it spurs me on to live my life as fully as possible. I focus on the beauty in my life and what I have now. I focus on the love I have and the joy and what having cancer has taught me – not on what I have lost, or what life would have been like if I'd been diagnosed much earlier. I feel I have been given another chance – it may be a shorter life than others, but by God, I intend to live it now. I have come to realise that cancer is not a death sentence but, rather, a catalyst for change.

I have had my down moments, of course I have, but I cannot say that I have had depression – despite all the drugs I am on that can cause this; neither have I put on weight which is another possible side-effect of the maintenance drugs that I continue to take. Again – that was a byproduct of a conscious decision to eat as healthily as possible – an alkaline and no sugar diet, which

I will discuss in a later chapter. I think I am fitter now than I have been in the last 10 years.

To sum up, the total faithful love and care that I have been given by those close around me has given me a feeling of worth that I never had deep down before. I know that I matter to people, I understand how important friendships are and I feel completely privileged and blessed to be alive and to have such a fantastic husband, family and network of friends.

Strangely enough, through my cancer I have discovered so much that is good about people. I have realised how true my friends and family are. I have been truly humbled by their acts of kindness, thoughts and empathy.

I have got so much closer to my girlfriends. Old friends who I hadn't seen in years came back into my life. It dawned on me then how lucky I was. These friendships hadn't changed in 30 years. You begin to appreciate so much the bonds of friendship. Humour plays a large part in these friendships too. I remember a very old friend coming to visit me in hospital after my triple lumpectomy and we laughed so much, I thought I was going to faint. We had tears rolling down our faces and the nurses came and joined in the party too. These are the people now that I know will be lifelong friends. We've all taken different paths in life and we may not see each other as often as we'd like to, but if it is a real and true friendship, time does not matter – you know they will always be there.

Many people want to help and just don't know how and some people say they want to but you are not sure if they really mean it. When they say, 'Let me know if I can help,' it was difficult to answer because I wasn't sure how much they were prepared to help and didn't want to put them in a difficult position.

There are some people who make the gesture to make themselves feel better and don't follow through. It was much easier when a person was a bit more forthright and actually suggested dates and times or asked me if I needed help with particular things – for example:

Have you got your school runs sorted? Leave it to me and I will sort out a rota
Give me a date to take you to chemo
Give me a shopping list for groceries
Are you covered for when you go into hospital? Could we have your children for some of the time or the duration?
I am going to the chemist/post office today, can I pick up/post anything for you?
I am free on Tuesday and Thursday, can I come and make you lunch?
I walk my dogs every Tuesday and Thursday nearby, could I walk yours too?
Why don't I come and water your greenhouse once a week?

I found that little routines and helpers naturally fell into place.

These are some of the things my friends have done for me, and this might give you an idea of what you can do:

- My mother-in-law lent us her flat in London for when I had my daily radiotherapy treatments, and a great friend who is a decorator helped us renovate it and made it lovely and cosy for me to recuperate. She gave her time for free and did not charge us any mark up on the things she bought. She also, with my cousin, had my children to stay for Easter so that my husband and I could go away – for a break between finishing chemo and having my mastectomy

- Christmas was looming and I was right in the middle of chemo and determined to give my children a perfect Christmas. A friend asked me if there was anything she could do to help on the practical side and I said that I didn't have a centre piece for the table. The next week the most beautiful centre piece you have ever seen arrived – my table was stunning, and all I had to do was put a few candles round. I still have it. I get it out every Christmas, and it reminds me of her and our bond of friendship

- My Christmas lights were broken – so another friend bought me some new ones
- A friend helped me decorate the house at Christmas and put up all the cards
- I was taken for walks
- I was helped with my errands
- My dogs were walked on a regular basis by a friend
- My children always had places to stay if I was too ill or had to be away. One friend took my daughter, Angelica every Tuesday night as that was 'chemo night' and I didn't want her to see me so unwell. For her, it was great – she had such fun on her regular sleepovers
- I was driven to and from radiotherapy and chemotherapy on a regular basis
- My parents came to see me often and made me lunch
- My sister who lived near me was always undertaking errands for me
- A group of my daughter's school mothers filled my freezer up with family meals for the children and healthy soups for me
- I was driven to school matches and other school events when I felt up to it
- My shopping was done for me
- I've a friend who is a wonderful cook who used to make me delicious treats that didn't have sugar in – and drop them round to my house

Along with the array of beautiful plants and flowers, here are some gifts that were so special to me, and helped me so much during my treatment:

- Several pairs of pyjamas, bed socks and a beautiful soft poncho
- Body creams, bath oils, hand lotions – all chemical- and paraban-free, of course. Parabens are chemicals that are widely used as preservatives by the pharmaceutical industry. They are cheap but very controversial because they have been found in breast cancer tumours, and they have been found to mimic oestrogen. The hormone oestrogen plays a role in some kinds of cancer. Indeed, my breast cancer is hormone positive
- Cosy hot water bottles
- Wheat or lavender pillows
- Lavender eye masks

Given that there are so many lovely gifts out there, it's better not to give chocolates, sweets or champagne – no matter how nice that feels. Sugar is the worst thing for cancer. It thrives on it. Best not to encourage it. However, one friend bought me some cupcakes in hospital and I just couldn't restrain myself! But I always say to myself you have to break the rules occasionally…

I found I wanted to surround myself with people who just 'were'. I found this out as my treatment panned out – different friends and family members were particularly helpful at different stages of my treatment. Some are great for chemo; some are great for doing errands – they all played a part. But the ones I found I wanted to give a wide berth were the ones who needed to be entertained!

It is very normal to be totally humbled by many of your friends and relatives who support you with wonderful gestures. Their love and support enthused me with a strength I didn't know I had, but sometimes I was taken by surprise by some people who knew what I was going through and acted as it they had no idea. These people were normally terrified. I learnt to try not to get upset by this behavior – it was *their* fear, not mine.

Very recently I sat next to a mother at one of my children's schools; she is a parent in the same year group – I barely knew her. We had a lovely time chatting and getting to know each other at lunch, and I was wondering why I didn't really know this lovely person, as I knew most of the parents in my child's year. After lunch she apologised profusely to me because she said that when she heard I had cancer she kept her distance as it frightened her so much. Her experiences of cancer were terrible and two people she had known well and been very close to had both died of cancer. She said she was happy we had now spoken because she was not so frightened any more and could see that, even if you are living with cancer, you can be a happy and normal person – and you are not going to die at any moment!

Sometimes if you are having a lot of treatment, it can go on for many, many months, like mine – years, in fact. It becomes part of your daily life – you just get on with it. Some people are surprised when you don't let them know that you are having another operation or, in my case, I got a nasty infection in my breast after my final breast reconstruction (16 months after diagnosis and many operations), and I was unexpectedly in hospital for a week right over the Easter period and unwell for weeks either side.

It was so exhausting, just re-arranging all the Easter holiday plans for my family and getting them looked after for those few weeks (my husband did an amazing job!) that I really didn't have the energy or time to let people know. The only people that knew were the people who happened to contact me during that period. Some people can feel quite miffed sometimes.

Once you are in the elite (ha ha!) world of cancer, procedures, scans and a host of other things that most people would be disturbed about become just everyday life to you. And sometimes, yes, you don't want to talk about it or you don't mention it because these things can take up so much of your life that you just don't have time and just want to get on with living. Intuitive people get that, yet they manage to acknowledge it at the same time which is of great comfort.

KEEPING CONTACT – WHAT'S BEST FOR EVERYONE?

I had no idea how tired I would get, and long phone calls were really not a good idea. It was helpful if people kept them to a minimum, but it's obviously important that you talk to your parents and family as much as possible – it's important that they are kept updated and know what's going on. They can be very supportive.

Group emails were a good way of giving information so that you don't have to be bothered all the time. The phone constantly going, the questions constantly being asked is seriously exhausting.

Texts were great. I often so much more appreciated getting these, rather than a call. It meant that I could reply when I felt ready and wasn't totally exhausted – sometimes I felt so unwell but found it hard to say: 'I'm sorry but I can't talk now.' It was difficult if somebody I hadn't seen for a while called – I didn't want to sound rude. I used to get really overwrought and stressed because sometimes I'd get five or six calls a day and if you figure you spent 20 minutes on the phone per person that's a lot of time when you're feeling very weak and supposed to be resting. I loved getting cards (especially with 'no need to reply' so no pressure!) – I kept them all in a box and, when I got stronger, I started to reply.

I could always do it when I felt strong. They were wonderful to receive, popping up on my screen – these wonderful messages from friends.

ACKNOWLEDGING THE SITUATION

I feel very strongly about this topic of emotional well-being. I have had endless chats with people who have cancer, or spouses or close relatives of people who have cancer – and we all have the same take on it. Without going into too much detail, the bottom line is please, please *acknowledge* the situation! It is about listening to what it is really real with grace and tact. I think this is the single most important thing to come out of this chapter. You can do this in many different ways. By acknowledging, you are immediately removing the elephant from the room.

I can think of many incidences that left me very upset and disturbed when my cancer was not acknowledged. People do this out of denial and fear – they don't know how to react. Here is one example – I had finished chemo, had had a bunch of operations, and was halfway through my radiotherapy. I was physically incredibly weak. I was aching all over and I made an appointment to have a gentle massage at my hairdresser – the hairdresser that I have been going to and been loyal to for 16 years (except for the previous few months obviously); God knows how much money I have spent there! I walked into the very large salon and there were all the regular stylists cutting and blow drying hair – all the people that I had bantered with for 16 years. Now, I know for a fact they all knew I was extremely ill because a friend had told me they'd all been talking about it. I walked across the floor and everybody kept their heads down or turned away, including the owner. It went eerily quiet except for the whirring hum of the hairdryers. I was so shocked. I went into the treatment room and undressed. The therapist said nothing either – even when I took my wig off and revealed my bald head. She said, 'Are you all right?' And I answered no not really – and she said banally, 'Don't worry, you'll be better soon.' I couldn't wait for it to be over. I cried, I got up to leave – I couldn't stand it and I couldn't stand the thought of running the gauntlet through the large salon to get out.

I guess I have to feel sorry for them – that they are all so full of their own fear they couldn't just say, 'Hello. I'm so sorry to hear what you're going through.' That is all I mean by acknowledgement. I didn't want pity, or to talk about it – just acknowledgment. It takes two seconds. I would have felt so much better.

Acknowledgment doesn't have to take the form of words either – it can be actions. I remember having dinner with another couple. The husband I hadn't seen for ages and am not particularly close to, but I am very good friends with his wife. When I walked into the restaurant, he got up and embraced me – not just the usual perfunctory double kiss on the cheek, but he took me by the arms, held me tight and hugged. That, combined with the look in his eyes, meant so much more than words. We didn't talk about my cancer at all that night – we didn't need to; it had been acknowledged and I was feeling greatly comforted. We went on to have a really fun dinner and stayed out far too late…

SOCIALISING AND GOING OUT

I limited socialising to only friends I was really close to for the first year and a half of my cancer treatment, with a few exceptions. My close friends were my cocoon of protection if we were in a restaurant. Meals were quick and I went home early, but I really enjoyed it – it was lovely to be out of the treatment and resting atmosphere and with my friends. Bumping into contemporaries was tough but I learnt how to handle it. I didn't go to any parties except for two. And these were very late on in my treatment, during radiotherapy. They were two very close friends celebrating two very important birthdays and they really wanted me there. They made a big effort to sit me next to someone I would know and not feel intimidated.

I remembered being quite anxious about how my contemporaries would react to me. I looked very different, my hair (wig) was a massive change, and I had lost a lot of weight. I remember being so tired and weak that I could barely stand up, but of course most people there did not realise that and I slightly wondered why I had come. Although I felt a bit like a rabbit in the headlights, it was a mixed experience, but mostly happy and positive. I certainly wouldn't have gone to any more, though. Those two were enough. With a big party you don't know who you are going to sit next to – so it is quite a lottery. I would spend the whole time asking my neighbor questions and getting them to talk about themselves to avoid talking about me. And when the inevitable question came – 'So what do you do?' – I didn't really know what to say. You have two choices: do you ruin their evening by telling the truth or do you say 'Nothing' or 'I am just a housewife/mother/partner'? It was hard for me to say this because it was so not me. I am a doer and along with my children and my home and family, my work, Lovedean, was a huge part of my life. I suppose my other choice was, 'Well, I was a successful business woman until last year when I was diagnosed with stage 4 cancer, so now I am being treated for it and that is what I do.' That would have made most people very uncomfortable.

I did, however, do something I had longed to do. I went with a friend to an art exhibition that I really did not want to miss. She understood my situation, so we agreed that we would 'whizz' round it – better to see it quickly than not at all. We did just that in 20 minutes, then went across the road for an absolutely delicious lunch at my favourite restaurant, where we were joined by our husbands. It was all carefully managed and a truly wonderful few hours – my great escape!

JUST BECAUSE I LOOK WELL DOESN'T MEAN I AM

On the assumption that my energies would be totally depleted, or that I may bump into someone I didn't know very well and there might be an awkward situation, I didn't socialise much at all. Even now, I am still careful about what invitations I accept. I make sure I don't go to bed too late and I leave when I am tired, because I know that tiredness and lack of sleep has a huge impact on staying well.

Even when people know I am being treated for stage 4 breast cancer, when they know it is technically incurable, they still can't comprehend that that is the case. They say, 'Wow – you look great. All better now, I see. Are you going to start your business again?' They would say, and still do say, 'Hello, you look great. So you're much better then? Are you getting on with life again?' ('Getting on with life?' Oh goodness – what do you think I've been doing for the last few years?)

These comments used to make me so angry. I always managed to look OK during my treatments – with a good wig, and by applying a bit of make-up, and making an effort with my clothes. And it was quite staggering how people assumed you were well or 'cured'. One remark was so awful I just had to laugh: 'Nobody feels sorry for you because you look so well!' Hmm.

Did I ever want to be felt sorry for? No. Did I want pity? No. Did I want empathy, understanding and acknowledgement? Yes.

I have learnt to respond without getting upset now, but initially it used to really bother me and make me quite upset. Because people generally want good news – they can be blind to reality if they want to be. My response to them is to generally to tell the truth in a clear, concise way; explain that staying well is pretty much a full-time job, that I still undergo a very light non-toxic form of chemo and bone treatments intravenously every three weeks – which leaves me a little off-colour; that I may be partaking in trials and so forth; that more surgeries are looming – and then I change the subject (hoping that they've taken it on board).

By being realistic about my situation I have been able to cope with it. So I would answer that no, I wasn't better – I wasn't well, I was still being treated, but was definitely 'getting on with my life', and happy too! They would sometimes still answer, 'But you must be better because you look great!'

So, you are never going to stop these things occurring – but I hope it's some comfort to know that it happens to us all. And if you are forewarned, then perhaps you will be better equipped to deal with it than I was initially. My advice: take a deep breath and try and let go of any anger welling up. Remember, anger is a negative energy; anger leads to stress – and there is no room for stress in your life.

Here is another story about how difficult people find it to acknowledge difficult circumstances: when I was very sick, having radical chemotherapy on a weekly basis for 24 weeks, I had had a routine CT/PET scan and MRI to see how the treatment was doing. We had wonderful news – *relatively* – which was that the tumours were showing signs of shrinking. This is the news that the oncologist expects as that is why I am being given chemotherapy in the first place. Nonetheless, obviously, my husband and I were really, really pleased that things were going in the right direction and we told people very close to us. We were clear and concise – there was nothing we said that could be misconstrued – yet a few days later I got two or three letters congratulating me on being cured and how wonderful to be able to start a new life.

I was devastated. How could these seemingly intelligent people have allowed something to be so wildly off the mark. I wanted to ring them and say, 'No, you dimwit! My tumours are responding to the chemo – that is all. That is what they are supposed to be doing! I am not cured, I will never be cured – I haven't finished my chemo; I haven't even started radiotherapy; I've only had two operations; I haven't had my triple lumpectomy; I haven't had my shoulder operation...' (And I could have gone on, if only I had known what was to come.) 'I haven't had my liver operation; I haven't had my mastectomy; I haven't had my fat cell transfer; I haven't had my reconstruction; I've got months of full-on treatment ahead.'

This happened frequently at other stages of my treatment, so in the end I stopped filling people in on test results verbally. It was too painful to experience the misinterpretations. Instead, my darling husband wrote very simple emails summing up everything.

I would find that people would look at me in surprise as I carried on normal life in the moments when I could. Life does not stop – it goes on. If I was doing the grocery shopping or errands in my local town people would think that I was better because I was out and about. Of course, this wasn't true. Just because I behave normally doesn't mean I'm OK. My grocery shopping was probably the only thing I was able to do in a day.

PEOPLE TO KEEP AT ARM'S LENGTH

During my new life, living with cancer, I have really come to know what a narcissist is. You must learn to recognise them because they can be very draining. The signs to look for are when your illness is actually centred around them, and what a terrible effect it is having on *them* and how difficult *they* are finding it to cope – with lots of tears and melodramatics! They want you to get better *their* way and do not support the way you are dealing with the disease. These people should have a Health Warning written all over them. You don't want to end up looking after these types emotionally – you must not let this happen.

I have often been stunned through conversations when the narcissists have gone on and on about their many ailments – which, by the way, they have the absolute right to do, but please: not every minute of the day! I would find it extraordinary that they could be so insensitive. I have often, for example, been around chat about the menopause: discussions about how people think it is creeping up on them, how they get hot flushes. I think to myself, wow, if only they knew. For me, instead of menopause creeping up I literally crashed violently into it overnight – due to the chemotherapy and other drugs administered. Not only that, but it goes on for months, even years. It's not nice, but you just deal with it; wear lots of loose layers so that you can strip off at a moment's notice. The worst thing is that you cannot do much to relieve the symptoms. You cannot take HRT (certainly for my type of cancer) like everybody else can. On this subject, I don't really join in, because if I revealed the type of aggressive and lengthened menopause I experienced – and still do – I'd feel that I was belittling their experience, which is also real and very unpleasant. Time to keep quiet on this one, and nod understandingly.

It is another difficult balance to strike, because you do, or at least I really did, want to know about other people's ailments and problems and be able to be understanding and provide an ear. Some friends would so thoughtfully go out of their way not to talk about their problems, and some would never stop.

There are also the people who just totally lack empathy. You soon work out who they are – they are incapable of understanding really what you are going through. Apart from the empathy-lacking part, they sometimes also seem to believe that you are simply trying to draw attention to yourself – and so they treat you as if you just have a bad cold. One adult who came to visit me in chemo actually asked me if cancer was contagious! I dine out on this story. They continued to ask me which 'hurt' more – chemotherapy or radiotherapy. This person wouldn't stop until I answered this impossible question.

It's best to avoid these people as it can be so upsetting, or make sure there is another person with you. Having this illness teaches you a lot about other people.

'WE'RE ALL GOING TO DIE ONE DAY'

Along with a lack of acknowledgement, the other terrible thing that fellow cancerites bring up is this supposedly comforting but totally ignorant comment that people make: 'We are all going to die one day, I might walk out of this door and get run over by a bus.' How many times have I heard this? Too many!

This is probably one of the most un-comforting things anybody could say. What they are actually doing is belittling your illness and all the strength you have put into your treatments and recovery. It is like a dagger through your heart. You realise that they have absolutely no idea what you have been through. Again – stay clear.

THE ENCOURAGING ONES WHO COMPARE YOU TO OTHERS

I think this response comes up level with the lack of acknowledgment. Urgh – this has happened countless, countless times. Now, I'm pretty much immune to it and I actually start laughing – which I guess is much better than before, when I would

p with anger and frustration. It hap-
s:

Helpful Person (HP):'My friend's mother had breast cancer and she's fine now. It's amazing what drugs they can come up with now. You'll be fine.' Well, that is like having a triple dagger rammed through your body!

Me:'Oh, really? What type of breast cancer did your friend's mother have?'

HP:'Oh, I don't know.'

Me:'What stage was her cancer?'

HP:'Oh, I don't know that either.'

Me:'Had it metastasised?'

HP:'Haven't got a clue, but she's fine now.'

Me:'How long ago was that?'

HP:'Don't really know. About five or six years.'

Me:'Did you know that there are many, many types of breast cancer, with varying stages of severity?'

HP:'No.'

Me:'Well, I am very happy for your friend's mother that she is now well; however, every cancer is completely different, so it really is irrelevant to me.'

And, of course, I want to say: 'How do you know I will be fine; can you see in to the future?'

What I really should have done when this first started happening – and do now – is fast-forward to the last line and cut out the dialogue. But this is really something that upsets people in our situation. Again, it is just people trying to be helpful, not knowing what to say, wanting desperately for everything to be OK.

You have to be quite tough about this as it happens a lot and that's not easy when you're feeling very weak. It is really irksome as it somehow makes you feel that your cancer is being trivialised. If the same person persists in these approaches then you must just tell them not to compare as there is nothing to compare with.

You can console yourself, however, with the fact that they are just trying to make you and themselves feel better. People hate bad news and they tend not to listen when you tell them what is wrong with you. It always surprises me when I know I have told people in very ABC language about my condition and then they see me a few weeks later and say, 'All better now?' – as if I have had a bad dose of flu. If I answer, 'No, not really,' then they say, '"Well you must be, you look great!'

It's extraordinary; people think that in order to be really ill, you have to look really ill. I never looked really ill on the surface except perhaps when I took my wig or headgear off (see plate), so it was difficult for some people to comprehend what I went through and, indeed, what I am still going through.

THE IGNORANCE OF OTHERS

This is a tricky issue. When I get questions fired at me that I've answered a million times before, I try to remember that I wasn't always a 'cancer expert' either and I can't really expect everyone to know as much as I now do. I try not to get fed up when I have explained clearly and concisely what my condition is and yet I am still asked the same questions over and over again.

This is quite wearing and you have to master the art of changing the subject quite rapidly.

PEOPLE'S REACTIONS ONCE INVASIVE TREATMENT IS OVER

As I have said, once you are through the chemo, surgery and radiation, people may treat you like you are better. But, in fact, this can be the worst time. By this point you are exhausted, your body, stamina and emotions have been ravaged. It's like you've been on a super-fast fairground wheel that has just stopped and I found that this was the time that I tried to make sense of it all. I finally had time to think and re-flect on what I had been through. People aren't so all over you any more with the same sense of urgency to help – and sometimes you can feel quite lonely.

I remember that sense of loneliness when I had finished all the major treatment and was feeling ghastly, trying to rest in my house, while my children and husband were gadding around downstairs. Occasionally one or two of them would burst in and out for some reason or another without seemingly a care in the world – and I remember feeling very isolated. You are caught between shifting sands – you are not ill enough to be in bed, yet when you try and do a few errands etc. you feel completely bushed.

I tried to explain to my children, friends and family that this was the worst bit. I stuck an information leaflet up on the kitchen cabinet which explained the after-effects of radiotherapy, hoping that they would read it and see that the side-effects for all these treatments can go on for many months after they've finished.

You are probably more exhausted at this point than at any other point in your treatment, also because you will be trying to do more – and this will be compounded. You may be fed up with being 'ill' and then push yourself too much. I certainly did.

THE OTHER HALF

It was so touching to see how conscious my friends and family were about how my husband was faring. It is, of course, a dreadful time for spouses/partners too and they can often get forgotten. I thought it was really important to give him all the freedom he wanted or needed. I encourage him to go out, go to parties, go away for the odd weekend, take the kids skiing – it was good for him and them. I wanted them all to be as happy as they could be and I liked it when they went away, as I didn't have to keep up quite such a pretence. I didn't have to put my wig on, or my make up etc. Sometimes it was a relief.

When the initial stages of your treatment are over and you have time to actually sit and try and make sense of it all, you can feel quite a different person. Well, you *are* a different person. Things that you once accepted about a partner or spouse, or your children or friends might not now be acceptable to you. You realise how fragile and how important life is and now instead of just 'muddling on' and brushing away things that have irked you for years, you now will say no! I have certainly changed and I want to make the most of every day that I have – and this has changed my attitude profoundly. There are things that I don't accept any more, and I am fully aware that those around me have had to get used to this. It may take a bit of adjustment in those ensuing months, and you may want to go to counselling (I touch on this further on in the book) with or without your family – but everything should even itself out in the end.

4
Treatment and Tests

From my diary:

> *Yesterday was a hard day, but it was a whirlwind of decisions, probing, gathering data, researching the best possible treatment. I spoke to my parents several times and by the evening we were all very composed and positive. They had all cleared their diaries and commitments for the coming months which was very comforting to know. I felt that they felt better and had come through their first day of my cancer well.*

THE ADMINISTRATIVE NIGHTMARE

For things to go as smoothly as possible during treatment, you or your carer have to be on top of the administration. Having cancer is like having a job. There are never-ending check-ups, tests, pre-op procedures, and meetings with oncologists and surgeons to co-ordinate. If you want to make it work for you then you need to know, ideally and as often as possible, what appointments are going to be necessary and get them made in advance by about a month. You do this by asking the secretaries what appointments will need to be made prior to, let's say, your surgery. Or ask, when, after surgery, you will be required to have a scan or a check-up. If you pre-empt and book in advance, then you don't run the risk of being called up a few days before and being told you have to come in in the next few days to have a scan and not being given a convenient time. Always take a notebook to the meetings with your consultant. Once you've finished your meeting, you can be so overwhelmed with all the information that's thrown at you it can be hard to take it all in and remember.

This can all be very stressful. There are some things that simply cannot be worked out in advance, though, and you will understand what these things are when they come along. Things do change sometimes and so do appointments – so no matter how organised you are, you have to accept this.

THE ORDER OF TREATMENT

There are many types of each variety of cancer – no two cancers are alike – which means that no two treatments are alike. For example, there are many types of breast cancer and each of those types has subsets, and each of those subsets also have subsets.

Every cancer treatment is tailor-made to the individual patient, so, really, in this world there is no space for comparison.

In my case, because my cancer was so advanced, the doctors decided to give me chemotherapy first (to shrink the tumour before surgically removing it), breast surgery (to remove the tumours), radiotherapy (to mop up any leftover cancerous cells), and then a procedure on my liver to remove any leftover tumours there. So it is for this reason that I am going to write about those treatments in this particular order.

In other cases sometimes the surgery is done first, followed by chemo. Some people don't need chemo at all, and some people don't need chemo *and* radio. It is very different for everybody: an extremely important point to remember, which is addressed in a later chapter.

CALENDAR OF EVENTS

I thought it might be helpful to make a table of my particular calendar of events. Obviously, it is personalised to me, but it gives you an idea of what to prepare for.

Following on from this, I have regular check-ups and scans and continue my three-weekly treatment of a very low dose/non-toxic chemotherapy.

Nov 2011		
Nov 3rd 2011	1st Diagnosis	Breast Cancer
Nov 10th	2nd Diagnosis Biopsies, CT/PET & MRI	Stage 3 Breast Cancer
Nov 15th	3rd Diagnosis	Stage 4 Breast Cancer Metastasise to Bone & Liver
	Port Fitted (see Page X)	General Anaesthetic
Dec 3rd		Weekly chemotherapy starts, until the end of March 2012
2012		
Jan 2012	CT/PET scans	
End of March 2012	CT/PET scans	Weekly chemotherapy ends
April 2012	Triple Lumpectomy	General Anaesthetic
	Giant Seroma excised – twice	
	Full Radical Mastectomy & Extender fitted	General Anaesthetic
May 2012	Unrelated shoulder operation	General Anaesthetic
June 2012		3 weekly intravenous treatment of Herceptin & Zometa start for foreseeable future
June 2012		Daily Radiotherapy starts for 6 weeks
June 2012	CT/PET Scans	
End of July	Liver Ablation surgery	General Anaesthetic
Nov 2012	CT/PET Scans	
Nov 2012	Coleman Fat Transfer	General Anaesthetic
March 2013	Full Breast Reconstruction	General Anaesthetic
April 2013	Week long hospital Admittance due to infection	Intravenous drip for 7 days

SCANS AND TESTS

CT/PET SCANS

You will have CT/PET scans soon after you are diagnosed and then either during or at the end of your treatment. I strongly advise you to determine from your oncologist when and how often he thinks you will need them. As I mentioned earlier, if you have this information to hand, then you can have a say in when they are booked – rather than have their office call you with some random date at short notice which may be hard for you to get to. Organising your scans at a time to suit you makes everything much less tiring.

A CT/PET normally takes up to three hours. It's important to know this so that you can plan your day, as they are quite tiring, especially if you live far away and/or have family to work around. And with some of the scans you have to fast for six hours – so do take this into consideration too.

A CT/PET scan is a combination of two scans.

- A CT scan (CAT scan) is a procedure that makes a series of detailed pictures of areas inside the body, taken from different angles. The pictures are made by a computer linked to an x-ray machine. A dye (contrast) may be injected into a vein or swallowed to help the organs or tissues show up more clearly. You can see lesions and anything that is not normal. It gives anatomical information, highlighting the soft tissues from the bones and will show anything that is unusual.

- A PET scan (positron emission tomography scan) is a procedure to find malignant tumour cells in the body. A small amount of radioactive glucose (sugar) is injected into a vein. The PET scanner rotates around the body and makes a picture of where glucose is being used in the body. Malignant tumour cells show up brighter in the picture because they are more active and take up more glucose than normal cells do. This enables the diagnosis of any disease in its early stage

Both these scans help your doctors to decide which treatment you need and also see whether your current treatment is working.

HAVING A CT/PET SCAN

Your doctor or radiographer will give you instructions about preparing for your scan. Usually you should not have anything to eat for six hours beforehand – good to know about this – so again you can schedule it to suit you.

On arrival you change into a hospital dressing gown and slippers. The radiographer puts a small tube (cannula) into one of the veins in your arm or the back of your hand to prepare you for the two different injections. After the first scan you have to lie still for at least one hour before commencing the second scan. They give you music to listen to in a quiet room, but they ask you not to move much so that the drug can be distributed evenly. Bringing in an iPod is a good idea – then you can choose to listen to your own music. I got rather bored of the 1970s selection the hospital provided and having to listen to them over and over again!

I found that I was always freezing when having these scans, especially once my treatment got underway. The rooms are very cold (to stop the machinery from overheating). Don't be afraid to ask for several blankets as they normally only give you one. And what they don't tell you is that you are often allowed to wear socks and a scarf. This helped enormously to keep me warm.

For the scan, you lie on your back on a narrow bed that moves through the scanner. The radiographer controls the scan from outside the room. During the scan they can see and talk to you. You need to lie as still as possible for 30 to 60 minutes while you have the scan. It is not painful, and there is a buzzer to call the staff if you need to.

Once the scans are over you can go home straight away. You need to stay away from children and pregnant mothers for the rest of the day so you don't expose them to any radiation (another reason to schedule this to suit you), although the dose is extremely small.

So, to recap – don't forget to:

1. *Organise* the scans to suit your schedule (in advance if possible). I prefer to make them early in the morning so that I am asleep for the starvation period – you are normally ravenous! Or make them at lunch time so that I can get up early and have a big breakfast at least six hours before. Then I get a friend to pick me up and we go and have a slap up afternoon tea. I always try to turn a horrible event into a nice one. I feel I've earned it!
2. *Fast* for six hours prior to the scan, if necessary
3. *Bring* a woolly hat, scarf, socks and iPod
4. *Bank* on the whole process taking three hours

MRI SCANS
(MAGNETIC RESONANCE IMAGING)

Depending on your diagnosis, you may also have an MRI scan prior to treatment, and every three months subsequently, or as often as the doctors think necessary – perhaps every six months, similar to the PET/CT scans.

This scan can take up to two hours, so again it is very important that you schedule this to fit around your diary. I have my PET/CTs and MRIs on the same day – which is extremely tiring, but I like to get it over and done with. This always suited me better, but that is not the best for everybody, of course.

MRI stands for Magnetic Resonance Imaging. An MRI scan uses magnetism and radio waves to build up a picture of the inside of the body. It can show how deeply a tumour has grown into body tissues. In other words, it is a means of 'seeing' inside the body.

The scanner is a large machine with a doughnut shaped hole with a padded bed which you are placed in. You can't feel anything when you are having the scan but the scanner is very noisy. It can feel claustrophobic, but you can stop the process any time you like. You will be given headphones to protect your ears and to listen to music, but you don't hear the music very well because of the noise the machine makes! Again, follow my previous advice about keeping warm.

The powerful magnetic field of the scanner can attract certain metallic objects, causing them to move suddenly and with great force towards the centre of the scanner. This can be extremely

CANCER IS MY TEACHER

dangerous. It is vital that you remove metallic objects in advance, including hearing aids, piercings, watches, jewelry, and items of clothing that have metallic threads or fasteners. There is supposed to be a system in place to ensure that you have removed all these things but the following happened to me and I was extremely lucky to get away with a minor injury.

I arrived to have an MRI on my brain – a false alarm, thank goodness! My mind was elsewhere as it was the eve before my final (hopefully) breast reconstruction and I was quite worried.

I took everything off, including my hearing aids (nothing to do with my cancer). The nurses gave me a metal key to lock away all my possessions and I put the key in my dressing gown pocket as there was nowhere else to put it. I was intending to remove it when I went into the scanning room – but after a wait of quite a few minutes, I clean forgot all about it (a symptom of 'chemo brain', covered later on). The nurses were supposed to check my dressing gown (a strict procedure) but they didn't and I went unwittingly into the scanner with the metal key in my pocket. As it was a brain scan, I was wearing a special helmet which proved to be my saviour. The key flew up along my body and jammed itself into my helmet and lodged itself quite powerfully in between the helmet and

56

my eyebrow, skimming my chin and causing grazing. It was all quite painful, but could have been much worse. It could have taken my eye out or sliced through my head.

So there is definitely a lesson to be learned here: always familiarise yourself with safety procedures and make sure they are being followed.

Here is a check list to go over things that may not enter into the screening room:

- Purse, wallet, money clip, credit cards, cards with magnetic strips
- Electronic devices such as beepers or cell phones
- Hearing aids
- Metal jewellery, watches
- Pens, paper clips, keys, coins, hairpins
- Any article of clothing that has a metal zip, buttons, snaps, hooks
- Underwires, or metal threads
- Shoes, belt buckles, safety pins

Check with the MRI technologist or radiologist at the MRI centre if you have questions or concerns about any implanted object or health condition that could impact the MRI procedure. For example, as I had a Portocath I had to let them know and get clearance.

Here is a checklist of things that may affect your eligibility to have an MRI and you must check with your doctor before and let the screeners know:

- Pacemaker
- Implantable cardioverter defibrillator (ICD)
- Neurostimulator
- Aneurysm clip
- Metal implant
- Implanted drug infusion device
- Foreign metal objects, especially if in or near the eye
- Shrapnel or bullet wounds
- Permanent cosmetics or tattoos
- Dentures/teeth with magnetic keepers
- Other implants that involve magnets
- Medication patch (i.e. transdermal patch) that contains metal foil

For some MRI studies, a dye (contrast agent) may be injected into a vein to help obtain a clearer picture of the area being examined.

The most important thing for the patient to do is to relax and lie still. Most MRI exams take between 15 and 45 minutes to complete, depending on the body part imaged and how many images are needed, although some may take sixty minutes or longer. You'll be told ahead of time just how long your scan is expected to take.

You will be asked to remain perfectly still during the time the imaging takes place, but between sequences some minor movement may be allowed. When the MRI procedure begins, you may breathe normally; however, for certain examinations it may be necessary for you to hold your breath for a short period of time. During your MRI examination, the MRI system operator will be able to speak to you, hear you, and observe you at all times. Consult the scanner operator if you have any questions or feel anything unusual.

When your PET/CT and MRIs are over, the images will be sent to your medical team. This normally happens quickly, and you will have made an appointment to discuss the results.

MRSA SWABS

You will be given regular tests for MRSA which is done by taking a swab from your nose.

ECHO CARDIOGRAMS

Depending on what cancer you have and the type of treatment, you may have to have an Echo Cardiogram every three months. I have to have this because I am on a drug called Herceptin, which works well for hormone-positive breast cancers. Herceptin can affect your heart muscle, although it is unlikely.

This procedure is totally non invasive. It is like having an ultrasound (which most women who have been pregnant will know all about) and takes about 15 minutes.

ULTRASOUND

An ultrasound is a procedure in which high-energy sound waves (ultrasound) are bounced off internal tissues or organs and make echoes. The echoes form a picture of body tissues called a sonogram. The picture can be printed to be looked at later.

GENETIC TESTING

Genetic testing is a very large and complicated subject. Although cancer is a common disease, only a fraction of all cancers are due to a mutation in an inherited gene. Genes are pieces of the DNA code that we inherit from both parents, and they usually work to protect against cancer. But if you have a gene mutation it means you have a high risk of developing breast and ovarian cancer.

In breast cancer, BRCA1 and BRCA2 are the two known genes that influence whether or not you are likely to get the disease. Women with a BRCA1 mutation have an estimated breast cancer risk of between 60 and 90 per cent, mainly between the ages of 30 and 80. Their ovarian risk is estimated to be between 10 and 30 per cent after the age of 50. A man with a BRCA2 gene mutation may have a 5 to 10 per cent risk of breast cancer and a 20 to 25 per cent risk of prostate cancer over a lifetime. If a woman is found to have the BRCA gene mutation, that would mean that each of her children would carry a 50 per cent chance of inheriting the gene.

If you are concerned about your family's history of cancer, you will be sent to a genetic specialist who will explain to you in great detail whether or not you are eligible for testing. Before you are seen, you will have been given a detailed family history questionnaire to complete at home. The specialist will look very carefully at this and then follow up with a phone call. At this point the specialist will decide whether or not you need to come in for an appointment to explore further whether you should have the actual genetics test.

Some cancer patients will be automatically recommended for genetic testing by their surgeon or oncologist due to the type of cancer they have. The outcome of the test will in turn help the surgeon decide on what type of surgery to perform – in the case of breast cancer, whether a double or a single mastectomy is appropriate.

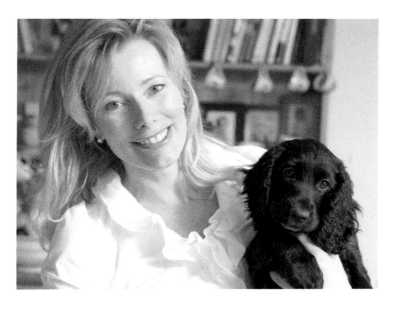

A couple of years before diagnosis – blissfully unaware
that my tumours had most likely taken root.

A few weeks after I started chemo. My hair started to fall out in clumps so I had it cut short

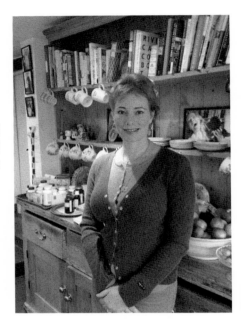

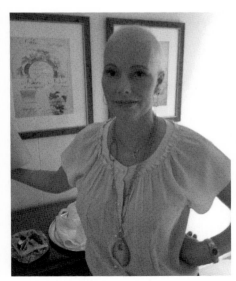

My hair didn't last long. My brother, Andy, shaved off the remaining clumps. I'm utterly exhausted here! And you can see the effect of the tattoos on my eyebrows

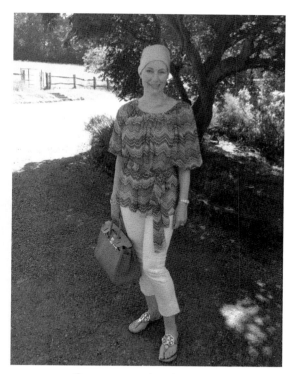

On my way to chemo –
this orange bandana was a particular favourite of mine in hot weather

With my husband. One of my turbans I had made out of a pashmina – very warm indeed for those freezing cold days

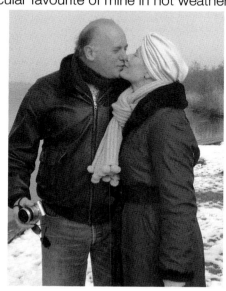

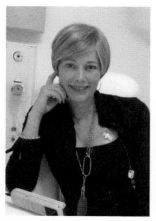
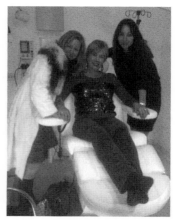

In chemo. I tried to make an effort as much as possible. I'd meet friends for lunch before and then bring them back with me. It kept my spirits up (note – you can see my port, top left)

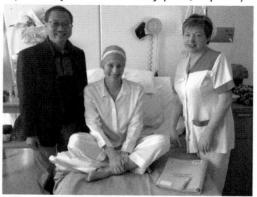

The next day, after my mastectomy –
with my breast surgeon Gerald Gui and my nurse

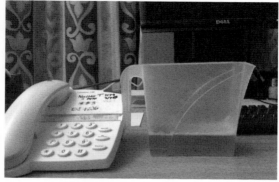

This was the amount of fluid that was drained from my seroma – ouch!

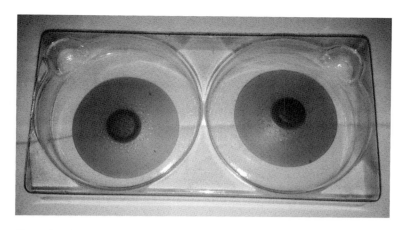

Prosthetic nipples. If your nipple(s) has/ve been removed, these are great to use until reconstruction

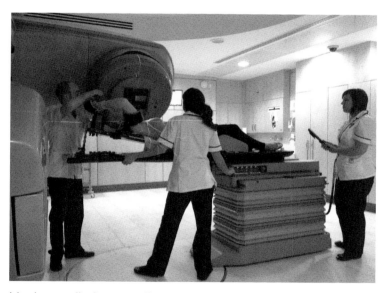

Having radiotherapy. I'm strapped in, and freezing cold. I mustn't move for the duration. My arm aches dreadfully, as it's my operated side that's being pulled back. The lights are the lasers they're using to line me up to the exact position for treatment. I find 'Mindfulness' really helps here...

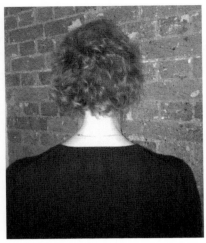

(Before)

Hair regrowth. A friend diplomatically pointed out to me that my hair was really out of control. Time to get the scissors out. Not a good look at all! (This was about six months after the end of chemo)

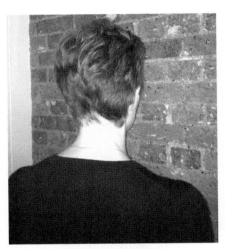

(After)

Chop chop: what a difference a good haircut makes. I found out that the secret is to keep chopping on a regular basis until the hair quality and growth normalises. Then you can grow it…

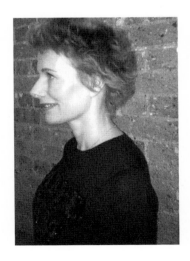

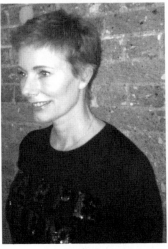

(Before)

(After)

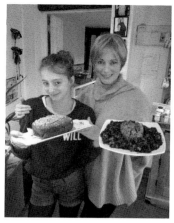

Eating well: cooking healthy food with my daughter, Angelica

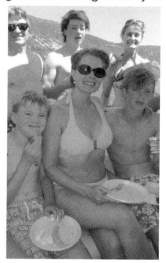

Three months after my full reconstruction. I don't think you can tell the difference

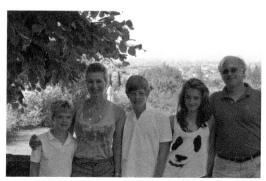

Ten months after diagnosis, we went on a family holiday to Italy to stay with friends

69

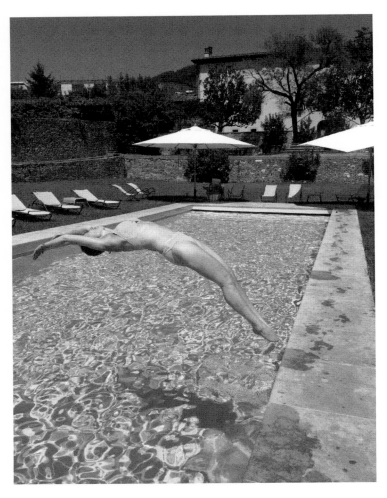

This was nine days after my liver operation and ten months since diagnosis. I was supposed to take it really, really easy. But as I walked past the pool, I had this yearning to do my party trick: a backward dive. I felt like a new person and it was a defining moment. I'd got through this much so far and I could still dive. I felt alive again! I felt normal…

5
Chemotherapy

Before I start on specific chemotherapy treatment, it is very important to stress the importance of good hygiene. When I started treatment I travelled with antibacterial gel and I made sure anybody who came near me used it – and I still do. I encourage my children to use it all times, and I instruct people not to come near me if they have a cold. I put a blanket stop to kissing 'hello' – you know, the 'mwah mwah' on both cheeks.

I also explained this to my children's schools. I did not want my children coming back home and giving me all sorts of bugs that would affect my treatment. The schools were very diligent about putting into practice my requests, which were that my children put on antibacterial hand gel several times during the day. In fact, now, I think one of the school's policies is now to have hand gel on the entrance to the dining room. My children themselves were very aware, too, and they kept a little bottle of it in their desks and school bags. I also gave them immune boosting supplements.

The last thing you want is to come down with a cold or an infection. This could interrupt your chemo and that becomes a real pain.

THE TREATMENT

So, chemotherapy is the use of medicines to kill or slow the growth of rapidly multiplying cells (cancer). It usually includes a combination of medicines, since this is more effective than a single medicine given alone. There are many medicine combinations used.

Chemotherapy medicines are given intravenously or orally. Once the medicines enter the bloodstream, they travel to all parts of the body in order to reach cancer cells that may have spread beyond the primary cancer. Chemotherapy is given in cycles of treatment followed by a recovery period. The entire chemotherapy treatment generally lasts several months to one year, depending on the type of medicines given, and what stage the cancer is.

THINGS TO DO BEFORE YOU START CHEMOTHERAPY

SEE A DENTIST

Your teeth and gums must be healthy before you start chemo. And it is a good idea to see the hygienist too as you will not be able to do that during chemo.

THINK ABOUT WIGS, HATS AND OTHER HEADGEAR

If you're undergoing the type of chemotherapy that may make you lose your hair, go and find your wig now.

You want to eliminate all your errands and have completed as many preparations as possible before starting chemo, as you will have so much on your plate already and will be starting to feel exhausted. I used a variety of all headgear – depending on the weather, location and how I felt.

You have a choice about your wigs. You can buy a real hair wig (very very expensive – £800-£1000) or a synthetic one (£50-£90). For me, the synthetic one was the no-brainer. Why would I want to spend time blow drying a real hair wig in my weakened state of chemotherapy? I loved my synthetic one. I could just put it on and there I was – perfect hair! I bought two wigs but actually only used the one I felt really comfortable with. Ironically, the one that I bought which was as close to my long blonde hair looked ridiculous on me and I looked and felt much better in the short zappy one!

Your hospital or cancer treatment centre will advise you on places close to you to get your wig, as will many other organisations some of which are listed in the back of this book.

The benefits of a wig:

- You never have to wash your hair
- Your never have to blow dry your hair
- Your hair is always healthy and shiny looking
- You never get greasy or knotty hair
- You barely ever have to brush your hair
- You never have a bad hair day
- You save a fortune not having to go to hairdresser

Maintenance was easy. I didn't bother with wig shampoos (more expense). I just washed it about once a week, very gently in shampoo mixed with a little conditioner in warm water. Then I let it dry overnight naturally.

I wouldn't say I enjoyed this part of the process, but I didn't find it a ghastly experience. It was too superficial for me. A phrase that really does not sit well with me is, 'My hair defines me!' Honestly, there is a lot more to worry about than losing your hair. And it shouldn't be your hair that defines you; it should be your inner soul, your spirit, your strength and courage to get through this.

HATS

There are so many hats you can buy designed for covering up hair loss. I had many different types and it was quite fun building up a collection. Some of them even have fake fringes attached to them!

I had hats for the day and also thin little hats for night time. I found these invaluable because your head can get chilly at night.

BANDANAS AND TURBANS

I had several bandanas and turbans made. These also were a lifeline. Sometimes when it was really hot, I didn't want to wear my wig. I had about four bandanas and three ready-tied (you just slipped them on) turbans made in different colours and fabrics. The turbans were great for the evening and my wool ones were fantastic for very cold days when I was taken to see my children playing their football matches – a lot warmer than the wig (see plate)!

SWIMMING HATS

Swimming is a great exercise to take when having chemo if you are up to it.

I didn't want strangers to see my bald head when I went swimming and so I bought some wonderful 1960s American-style glam swimming hats. They were such fun and looked very classic. There are times when you want to forget you have cancer, and swimming is one. I didn't want the 'pity' look from strangers and the 'frightened' look from their children.

DEAL WITH THE EYEBROWS

I had my eyebrows tattooed within a few days of finding out I needed chemotherapy. Some beauty salons do this. For me, it was really important to look as normal as possible, so that I could feel good, confident and able to go about my business without that 'pity' or 'frightened' look I mentioned previously. Looking well makes those around you feel more comfortable.

I also had the upper lids of my eyes tattooed – this helped the loss of the eyelashes look much less apparent. If you don't tattoo, you can always just pencil them in with an eyebrow pencil and powder. These are useful too for when some hair starts to grow back – you can even the brows out.

GET A LAPTOP

If you do not have a laptop, I think it is a great investment. I found it much easier and more comfortable to do my admin from my bed, rather then come downstairs to my stand alone computer. I felt much too unwell. Then you can keep on top of things if you do a little every day, rather than put everything off because you are too ill to go downstairs. You want to make your environment as cosy as possible.

PERHAPS GET A PORT FITTED

A portocath (port) is a soft plastic tube tunnelled under the skin of the chest. The tip of the catheter lies in a large vein just above the heart and the other end connects with the port. Under the skin, the port has a septum through which drugs can be injected and blood samples can be drawn many times.

If you are going to have a port fitted, it will be done just before you start your treatment. I chose to have a port because I did not like the idea of having to be cannulised every time I went in for chemo, and I knew that in my case I would need it for many years to come. But most people's cancer is not at stage 4, and that means that you will only need to be cannulised for the duration of your treatment and not for the following maintenance treatment. The port has caused me no problems and I still use it for my intravenous infusions today. In fact, in the picture of me wearing the wig in chemo (see plate) you can see where the port is.

DECIDE ABOUT CHEMO BUDDIES

It is lovely having chemo buddies, but do not schedule in too many visitors. It becomes very wearing and tiring. You need to rest through these treatments, and keep as much strength as possible.

Make it a nice occasion. Try and have it at the same time – it makes it so much easier to organise. I always had it at 2.30 on a Tuesday, and I still do. (Although now it's every 3 weeks and it is a different type, a non-toxic sort – a maintenance treatment often given to patients with stage 4 cancer.)

I would meet a friend for lunch around the corner from my clinic, and then they would accompany me to chemo. They would stay with me for about an hour and a half, and then they would leave me so that I could have a rest.

Many cancer clinics offer complementary medicines, such as reflexology. I used to, and still do, have this during my rest in treatment. It is so wonderful that I fall asleep during it – very unusual for the insomniac me! After that, I would have a visitor for the last hour or so, and with that a nice cup of tea. If you are feeling completely rotten, then don't worry about cancelling your visitors – they will understand.

You will discover a true brand of 'angels' once you walk through the door of the chemotherapy unit. These nurses are totally dedicated, selfless, bright and smiley. If you arrive feeling rather ghastly, I can guarantee you will be feeling better once you see their faces. Their positivity and good cheer rubs off on you immediately. They are the most special people. I found it impossible to be down. I think I have only cried once during chemo and that was when my father and step-mother came with me, quite far down the line, and I saw the love and pain in his eyes and I could see he was bravely holding back his tears; he wasn't able to say goodbye because he was too upset and he didn't want me to see. Once they had left I cried too – the only time I have ever cried there. I couldn't bear the pain he was going through and bravely trying to disguise it.

Always make sure somebody picks you up afterwards and drives you home. It is important to be firm with your visitors and to give them times that they agree to stick to. You have to think from their point of view, they don't know what *you* want or how *you* are feeling, so if you let them know, they will be much happier too.

You may not feel much different after the first few sessions of chemo, but as they progress you start to feel more and more tired. Schedule in rests every day to suit you.

When you are actually resting, turn off the phones and computers. Even if you don't sleep (always an issue for me), you will have still done your body the world of good.

During chemo, I just could not drive, except for small distances. I felt too weak and as if my brain was not functioning properly. I felt unsafe most of the time.

I cannot stress enough: REST REST REST!

Accept help from other people. Everybody wants to help – whether it is school runs, shopping or cooking. Further on in this book I make a list of all the things I can think of that people did for me that I found helpful.

Think about getting a TV in your room or make sure your living room is nice and cosy for that. A lot of people find reading books quite difficult during chemo, and you may prefer to listen to the radio or watch TV. Book tapes are a great idea – you can catch up on all the classics you that you have always meant to read.

Try and take a little exercise every day. At first I did my usual dog walks, then they got shorter and shorter as my chemo progressed. I actually felt very unsteady on my feet. But my friends would come and collect me and take me on a short walk – it was so invigorating and so good for me to get fresh air and oxygenate the blood, and my dogs were happy too! I tried to do this every day. I also did simple yoga and when I was totally exhausted, I just did stretches in my bedroom.

YOUR FIRST DAY AT CHEMO

You arrive at the hospital/clinic. You are checked in and weighed so that they know how strong to make the chemotherapy medication. They will always keep a very close eye on your weight – for the medication, but also to make sure you are not losing too much. The medication is tailor made for you.

You will be given a little area which I liken to a 'pod' with a very comfortable bedlike chair (which you can lie almost flat if you prefer), where you can be private if you like, or leave the curtains open if you want to be in the fray. This will be your home for the next few hours, and next few weeks or months.

Ask for a blanket and a small pillow – it makes you feel much more cosy. Take your shoes off and put on some slippers or bed socks. Ask for water and make sure you drink a lot.

The nurse will go through a long list of questions about your general health. Questions such as: How are you bowels? Are you tired? Do you suffer from indigestion? At this point you must tell them exactly how you are feeling. It is very important, as then they will be able to give you all the medicines you require to counteract these symptoms. For example, if you have constipation (which you can get from the treatment) you must tell them. Always take medication at the first sign of the particular ailment, before it gets time to build up and get chronic. If the medicines don't work for you then tell the nurses, as there are lots of different types of medicines to counteract any particular ailment. It is all about communication and finding the right relief for you, and you may have to try several times, before you get it right.

The next step is blood tests. You can't start chemo without these results (so there will be a wait between the results coming through and starting chemo). The nurses have to make sure that your blood counts are OK. Ask for a full print out of your blood tests – it's always a good idea to have them at home to compare. Keep an eye on your glucose and cholesterol levels – your diet can greatly influence them.

Once blood tests come back and they are okay, then the chemo is ordered from the lab. While waiting for the chemo, they will cannulise you or gain access through your port.

Sometimes if your bloods are not good enough, they will not be able to give you chemo and you will have to have booster injections and come back later. This is why it is important to have a very healthy immune boosting diet (more of that in the next chapter), and to keep as well as possible. After this, they will hook you up to the machine and they will start with a saline flush, to flush the system, then there will be bags/pouches of various medications – steroids, antihistamine (to prevent allergic reactions), anti-sickness drugs, and the actual chemo medicine. One by one, these medicines will be administered over the course of several hours.

You are able to walk around and go to the bathroom because your IV is mobile and runs off a battery when unplugged. Just remember to plug it back in or the alarms will go off – I know from experience!

The nurses will check and monitor on you all the time.

There will be drinks and meals/snacks available. Try to eat healthily and drink LOTS of water. It is very important – you need to flush out the toxins.

Most units offer complementary therapy, such as reflexology. I found this very relaxing and it helped me to rest and alleviates anxiety. Afterwards you may feel a bit spaced out – this is why it is very important to have someone come and collect you.

On your first day you will leave which what feels like a suitcase of pills and medications to counteract any side effects.

YOUR CHEMO SURVIVAL KIT

Remember, you will be in your pod for several hours. When not resting, napping or having visitors you may want to bring other things in too, such as books, a laptop, etc. It's nice to have a choice of things and makes you feel more at home. I even bought pictures of my kids! The unit will have magazines and newspapers so you don't need to bring them.

- Bring in some bedsocks – you may get chilly staying still for so long, and the actual chemo can make you cold. It is nice to take your shoes off and cosy up
- A warm hat was essential for me. It was nice to take my wig off for the duration and let my head breathe
- Blankets and pillow – you will be provided with these, but of course you can bring your own if you prefer. I always bring a very soft poncho which is loose and comfortable but makes me feel snug and warm
- Facial spritzers, eye and nose lubricating drops – I always found my face eyes and nose felt very dry through the session, and afterwards

POSSIBLE SIDE-EFFECTS OF CHEMOTHERAPY AND HOW TO DEAL WITH THEM

Before reading this very long list of possible side-effects, please understand that not all of these will happen to you. And some of them will happen in a minor way and some a bit more severe. I may even have missed some out – but please remember that when you start chemo you will be given medication to counteract any harsh side-effects, and you are encouraged to take them.

The specific side-effects you will experience depend on the type and amount of medications you are given and how long you will be taking them. The most common temporary and remediable may include:

- Bone ache
- 'Chemo glow'
- Coldness
- Diarrhoea and/or constipation
- Dry eyes and blurred vision (blepharitis)
- Dry mouth
- Dry/sore nose
- Excess hair – or lack of!
- Fatigue
- Hair loss
- Heartburn
- Higher risk of infection

- Loss of appetite
- Memory loss i.e. 'chemo brain'
- Menopause and hot flushes
- Mouth: sore gums and teeth
- Nausea and vomiting
- Neuropathy (tingling hands and feet)
- Scalp irritation

Just to give you an idea, I suffered from hair loss (completely), menopause, mouth sores, dry skin, fuzzy brain feeling (otherwise known as 'chemo brain'), terribly dry eyes, a little nausea and bone ache and a huge amount of fatigue.

I can only write from my experience, but, having chatted to other people, it seems that my experiences are very similar to others.

Here are some ways of coping and dealing with the above side-effects, a lot of which I discovered 'along my journey':

BONE ACHE

Your oncologist will give you medication for this.

CHEMO GLOW

This isn't a myth – it really exists. My skin lost all its oiliness and I no longer had a shiny T-zone. My face became rather like porcelain. I reckon the chemo must have nuked all the bacteria – it was as clear as a bell!

People used to say to me, 'Gosh you look so well! I can't believe it. You look better than ever!' If only they had known. But I have to say it was a great confidence booster. A good wig, tattooed eyebrows – hey presto!

COLDNESS

You definitely feel the cold much more during chemo. This is when the warm hat comes in very useful.

DIARRHOEA AND CONSTIPATION

I got diarrhoea and constipation quite often, and sometimes very severely. Your body is very delicate at this point and you have to learn how much anti-diarrhoea medication to take and which type of treatment to use that suits you. Because your body is so fragile, sometimes it goes the other way and you then get acute constipation. You can find yourself rocking between the two.

After a while, I worked out which type of medicine to take and exactly how much to create the right balance.

DRY EYES (BLEPHARITIS)

I suffered from dry eye syndrome and occasionally got blepharitis. I used hydrating eye drops for these which relieved the dryness and irritation.

I used to put hot pads on my eyes morning and night, and then massage the lids. This would get all the tear ducts working and flowing again. I would use eye moisturizing sterile eye drops all the time. The trick is to keep the eye as moisturised as possible so that you don't get build up of debris which then blocks up the tear ducts and prevents them working. Sometimes the tear ducts can get infected because they are not working properly.

I also had blurred vision which is why I found it difficult to read lengthy books and watch television. My eyesight has deteriorated a little which I do put down to the chemo.

DRY MOUTH

Ask for a spray lubricant for your mouth. It really helps.

DRY/SORE NOSE

During chemo, if you lose your hair on your head, the chances are you may lose the hairs in your nose. And this in turn can give you a constant runny, sore, dry nose, which can, as in my case, lead to nose bleeds. A nasal moisturiser bought over the counter can really help with this.

DRY SKIN ON FACE

My face used to be combination type skin – slightly oily. Once the chemo got its grip on me, I noticed my skin getting less and less oily. All the impurities in my skin disappeared. Everybody said I looked years younger! I guess it's the chemo that is killing everything in your body. I also put it down to radically changing my diet, cutting out all sugar, dairy, alcohol and coffee – more about diet and nutrition later on.

I used to massage in facial oils every night, and tinted SPF moisturiser on my face during the day. It was great – I didn't have any shine on my skin during the day, something I had battled with for years. See Chemo Glow!

DRY SKIN ON YOUR BODY

Remember, your skin is your largest 'living' organ and it needs a great deal of care and attention when undergoing treatment. I strongly recommend that whatever you put on your skin is free from chemicals, especially parabens, and organic.

Your skin may get terribly dry. I used to slather myself with body, hand, face and foot cream all the time – of course, always with natural products. I always used lots of bath oil too.

My massage lady made me up concoctions of facial spritzers too – my face would sometimes feel so tight. There are so many different types you can get. During chemo I found them invaluable as my skin always felt so dry.

This all sounds rather laborious but it made a huge difference to my comfort.

EXCESS HAIR – OR LACK OF!

Rejoice, you won't have to wax or shave anything for the period you are having chemo!

And if you have radiotherapy around your armpit for breast cancer then you will have hardly any hair at the site ever. At least that's one armpit where you don't have to think about depilation…

FATIGUE
(NOT TO BE CONFUSED
WITH EVERYDAY TIREDNESS)

Nearly everybody who has chemotherapy has some fatigue. Everybody has tiredness but fatigue is something different. It is a relentless, whole-body tiredness, on a constant basis which is not cured by a good night's sleep and can be very hard for people around you to understand. And drawing from my own experience and the experiences of many contemporaries, the effects of the chemotherapy on the body can be of the most disturbing, unforgiving and life-interfering sort.

Of course whether or not you experience extreme fatigue will be down to a host of factors, some of which are listed below:

- You have very advanced cancer so your treatment is more radical
- Your immune system is low (due to your treatment)
- You may develop aenemia
- You are in pain
- You are reacting to other medications given to you whilst on chemo
- You are experiencing a range of emotions such as anxiety/stress or depression
- You are not sleeping
- You are experiencing hormonal changes
- You are not taking much exercise
- You are having trouble eating, or at least eating the *right* foods (diet is so important and there is a whole chapter on this later on)

The signs of fatigue are:

- Lack of energy
- Negative emotions and lack of interest in day-to-day activities

- Having a fuzzy brain, not being able to think clearly or make decisions
- Not being able to concentrate or focus on watching TV, reading and/or chatting to friends
- Breathlessness after small activities or jobs around the house
- Weakness, nervousness, anxiety or impatience

What can you do about fatigue?

First, you have to give in to it. As I said earlier, you must REST REST REST! – and you must ACCEPT ACCEPT ACCEPT! And in order to do this you must feel comfortable delegating tasks to friends and family.

I am harping on about this because it is pertinent for me – and I suspect many other people. I always take on more than I can do, so I am afraid I sometimes launch into doing too much. It happened quite a lot during radiotherapy. By this point I had endured eight surgical operations, radical chemo, radiotherapy, a mastectomy, a lumpectomy and much more, but I wasn't going to miss my children's sports days (three of them) or Archie's Holy Communion. The end of the summer term at school is always packed with events, speech days and so on. But yes, I did pay for it! The funny thing that I experienced with chemo and radio was that I would feel alright if I didn't exert much energy – so I would always assume I could do normal things and then, of course, I would find myself at a children's sports match, or in a supermarket in a desperate state of collapse and desperate to get home.

Prioritise on the important tasks to hand and set yourself very realistic goals. If you are like me and do a thousand and one things a day, it can be very demoralising to feel at the end of the day that you haven't achieved much. But actually, you have – you have taken care of yourself and are helping your body to recover and cope with the treatment and by extension you are helping those around you, who will be relieved see that you are probably coping and feeling better. You must alter your expectations entirely and then you won't feel let down.

HAIR LOSS

I started to lose my hair almost immediately. It started to come out in clumps in the shower. Three weeks into chemo, I realised it was time to get it cut into a really short sassy style (see plate)!

I hoped that I would be able to keep it for a while, but more and more fell out and that's when I realised that I would have to start wearing a wig or other head gear. But at least I got through a few weeks of having it. Eventually, I lost all my hair – my brother shaved off the last few tufts for me using a barber's electric razor. We did it on the spur of the moment; it was quite an intimate procedure and very poignant. I wasn't too alarmed as I knew this would happen, and I had already bought my wig. In a funny sense, I felt relieved because I no longer had to worry about my falling-out hair.

And there is nothing you can do about losing your lashes and brows – but as I mentioned earlier on, I tattooed both. This made a huge difference, and you honestly would not have noticed I didn't have them unless you looked very carefully. I managed to avoid that 'chemo' look. Though sometimes it did work to my disadvantage as people wouldn't believe that I was very unwell!

When your hair first starts growing back it can look quite odd. Mine came back slate grey, all soft and fluffy like a new born chicken, and it was quite patchy – it did not look very nice! So I used to keep wearing the bandanas/turbans/scarves/wigs when out and about. Then it went all wild, frizzy and mad scientist's look. A friend kindly pointed out that it should be cut again into a really sharp funky look to get through this period. When I saw the back of my head in the mirror I was horrified. I looked like an old granny! Once I had had it cut – it looked so much better (see plate).

As my hair came back, I used oils and masks on my head. I don't know whether they worked or not, but it made me feel good – and that can't be bad. I splashed on rosemary water on to my hair in the morning to try and tame it a bit. It is supposed to be very good for your hair and feels very refreshing.

The best way I found to get my hair looking good was to keep on cutting it. That would even out all the wispy bits. And only when I was happy with its texture did I start letting it grow longer. It's taken a long time, but two years later I love my new hair; it's thicker and glossy and looks much healthier than before. I don't put any colour or any products in it. It is 100% my natural colour. I never thought I'd ever like short hair!

THE COLD CAP
(ALSO KNOWN AS SCALP COOLING)

A cold cap can be used during some (but not all) chemotherapy treatments with the intention of helping to reduce hair loss from the head (it does not help other areas of the body such as eyelashes, eyebrows and pubic hair).

A very cold cap is literally placed on the head. As chemotherapy drugs are carried around the body via the bloodstream, the cold cap works by shrinking the small blood vessels that supply the hair follicles which means that less of the chemotherapy drugs will actually reach the follicles, and in turn less hair is likely to fall out.

In order for the cold cap to work, your scalp temperature needs to be kept low for the whole time the drugs are circulating in your blood, and it needs to be administered before your actual chemotherapy drugs are given (so you start with a cold head) and for a time afterwards. Consequently, this will lengthen your time in your clinic.

Cold caps are quite heavy to wear and cumbersome and also can make you feel rather chilly. I personally did not choose to have the cold cap because I wanted my treatments to be as comfortable, tolerable and quick as possible. Plus there is no guarantee that it will work and then you have gone through all that discomfort for nothing. I also felt that if it only reduced my hair loss, I would rather have no hair at all and fantastic head gear as opposed to straggly, thin bits of hair that were difficult to manage, looked unhealthy and gave me that 'victim' look!

HEARTBURN

Your oncologist will provide you with the correct medication for this. Eating an alkaline diet (which will also help keep you healthy and strong) will also help tremendously.

HIGHER RISK OF INFECTION

Because your immune system is taking such a battering with the chemotherapy drugs, you will be at a higher risk of infection. Be careful who you come into contact with, stay away from germs and keep eating that healthy diet (this is covered in a later chapter).

Other things you may not think about when trying to avoid infection:

- Wear gloves while doing housework or gardening
- Avoid cutting your cuticles when manicuring your nails. Use care when cutting your toenails
- Frequently wash your hands with soap and warm water especially before preparing food, and after using the bathroom or after touching soiled linens or clothes
- Protect your skin from scratches, sores, burns, and other irritations that might lead to infection. Use insect repellents to prevent bug bites
- Use antibacterial lotion on your hands and get your family and friends to do that too. I made everybody coming to visit me in chemo spray with antibacterial

LOSS OF APPETITE

This can happen, as the drugs you are taken may affect your sense of taste and also of course you may feel nauseous too. Hopefully the anti-nausea drugs will help you with your appetite, but please try and eat well and build yourself up.

MEMORY LOSS – I.E. 'CHEMO BRAIN'

This is very common and leads to difficulty in paying attention and managing day-to-day activities. It really can make you feel utterly helpless and hopeless sometimes.

People often notice these problems during chemotherapy treatment. Within one year of treatment, many people find these difficulties greatly improve or no longer exist. However, for some people, chemo brain can continue for years following completion of treatment. If you have chemo followed by radiotherapy, the effects can be more severe. I am still suffering greatly from memory loss. For example, I think I started driving much too early – there have been times when I didn't know where I was in the car (despite being somewhere local that I should have recognised). And another time, I went to see a fantastic film and a few days later I could not recall anything about it. I couldn't remember if I had actually seen the film or just seen the trailer! This obviously made me feel hopeless, frightened and panicky – it was uncharacteristic. It's quite difficult for other people to understand, because if you mention it, they often say, 'Oh yes I have that. It's just our age/the menopause...' – but what they don't realise is we are not talking about the same thing. It is completely different and much more severe.

MENOPAUSE AND HOT FLUSHES

I went hurtling into menopause shortly after starting chemo. This happened to me because I am being treated for 'oestrogen positive' breast cancer. So my chemo was a type of chemo that was taking away all the oestrogen in my body, very suddenly and very quickly. Not only was the chemo designed to rid my body of all oestrogen, but so were other medicines that I still take, such as Tamoxifen.

The major symptom of this was hot flushes and fluctuations in body temperature (which I still get to this very day). One minute I was boiling hot and shedding my clothes and the next minute freezing cold. At night it was the same – sometimes I would wake up totally soaked. My head would be damp and hot too. It's not that pleasant, but in the grand scheme of everything else that is happening to you it's just another side-effect that you learn to accept and deal with.

Wear lots of layers, then you can strip off accordingly. Obviously, unlike people who don't have cancer, you cannot take any medications to relieve it. No HRT! Or herbal remedies. I still have these symptoms but I've just got used to it.

MOUTH: SORE GUMS AND TEETH

A dry mouth is very unpleasant but quite common and can be easily remedied. Tell your chemo nurses and they will provide you with some drops or spray for your mouth. You can also buy special toothpaste and mouthwashes over the counter to help with this. It is not uncommon to get thrush in your mouth which is uncomfortable but treatable. It is quite common for teeth to become painful. You can get mousse type gel from your dentist to help with this.

Mouth ulcers are common too. I suffered from these. There are lots of fancy *expensive* products to alleviate these, but I preferred good old-fashioned gargling in salt water which does the job perfectly.

NAILS

These can become dry and flaky. To try to keep them in tip top condition, file them right down and massage nail oil into them as often as possible. I used to have very good nails, but I am afraid mine haven't recovered yet. If you want polish on them, there are now nail polishes out that are non-toxic.

Ask your beauty salon – it's not possible to find these in an ordinary chemist.

NAUSEA AND VOMITING

You will be given anti-sickness medication. You can also help by eating in small portions or nibbling throughout the day.

For some people it can be very debilitating. For me, it wasn't too bad.

NEUROPATHY
(TINGLING IN THE HANDS AND FEET)

If this happens, your oncologist will keep a very close on eye on it. It is very important that you let him/her know. A little tingling is OK, but if it gets unbearable you may have to change your chemo. I suffered mildly from this.

SCALP

Light head massages I found very relieving. I also used to put all sorts of masks and moisturising products (all natural, of course) on my scalp to help prevent it from drying out and getting itchy.

VULNERABILITY AND FRAGILITY

The list of possible side-effects from chemo is daunting, so I thought I would end this chapter on a more positive note. My experience of chemotherapy has left me with an important legacy, which concerns vulnerability and fragility.

As well as being primed for adversity, as I feel I have been, I feel also that when you have suffered a trauma as dramatic as this, you then become much more aware of other people's suffering. An illustration of this is when I went into my local town centre to do a few errands. I was right in the middle of my radical chemotherapy. I was very weak. But of course, I thought I was fine and drove in. By the time I had arrived and parked my car, I was completely shattered, dizzy and with blurred vision and excessive thirst. My legs felt like giving way and it was all I could do just to lift my bag off the car seat. But I was determined to do these few simple errands by myself.

I am normally a dreadful jay-walker. I usually run across the roads skimming in and out of traffic as I am too impatient to wait at crossings. Yes, I know – extremely dangerous! I've always done it and it's hard to change the habit of a life time. However, this was definitely not an option this time. I went to the traffic lights, and waited with everyone else to cross. The green light started flashing but I felt frightened and vulnerable. I couldn't judge the speed of the cars – I didn't feel like they were going to stop at the lights. I felt like I was in the chaos of Piccadilly Circus rather than the smaller quiet town of Haslemere.

It was then that I realised how truly vulnerable and frightened old people must feel. Now, whenever I see an old person crossing the road, or struggling with their shopping, I always try to help.

6
Surgery

There is something all cancer patients – and, indeed their friends and families – must understand and accept: operations may not always go as planned. You may have to have more than one operation, a 'tweaking' or 'fine tuning'; you may get an infection; you may not heal well. There are lots of factors that can influence these things and I think you have to go into this stage of treatment understanding that these things, however unlikely, could happen. Then, if they do, it is easier to handle and to get your head around. *Remember: procedures, results, assessments, decisions! One by one, step by step!*

My final outcome has been fantastic, but there were some hiccups along the way, as you will find out in this chapter.

I had a very advanced cancer that had spread and I presumed that I would have a mastectomy, but then when it came to making a decision, I was offered a triple lumpectomy with sentinel node removal (removing the sentinel node would enable the surgeons to see if my cancer had spread to my lymphatic system). I couldn't believe I was being offered a triple lumpectomy as opposed to a mastectomy – how could that be?

I was told that it may not be enough but that there was a jolly good chance of success. So I decided to go along with it – if there was a chance, I was going to go for it.

However, it turned out that the margins, or borders, of the tissue they removed were 'positive', suggesting that all of the cancer might not have been removed, so I had the full mastectomy 10 days later. I didn't feel bad or let down by this because my surgeon had clearly told me about the chances and I thought them worthwhile to take. It is quite common to blame your surgeon when things don't go according to plan – but this is pointless, so try not to! So you see, this illustrates the fact that situations can change. I went from mastectomy (horror) to lumpectomy (elation) to mastectomy (horror) in 10 days – quite a lot to get the head round.

Again, I will recount my own personal journey through surgery. Your experience will inevitably be different, but I hope the following will help.

A NOTE ON DECISIONS AND ACCEPTANCE

I nearly drove myself mad trying to decide whether or not to insist on having a double mastectomy. I saw my surgeon for progress meetings during my six months of chemotherapy. He did not want to commit to what sort of surgery he would be doing, he was sure that I would not need a double mastectomy – for very sound medical reasons. But I was exposed to so much general chit chat from well meaning, but medically ignorant people who all said that I must have both my breasts removed – how crazy I would be not to! I was constantly being told that other people had, even people who did not have breast cancer but who were at risk of it. I have come to think of this as the 'Angelina Jolie Effect' and it made sense to me too at that point. But I was ignorant at the time and I realised after a few months that they were wrong. Their reasoning was not based on medical facts, which also take into account a variety of complex issues. I understood much later on that if my surgeon thought that both my breasts should be removed he would have told me! After all, we both wanted the best outcome. I wish now that I had accepted that sooner.

I wasted so much angst on this subject and so much energy trudging round to other surgeons getting second opinions, and endlessly discussing it with friends and other breast cancer patients who had had singles or doubles, trying to work out the pros and cons; the 'whys' and 'ifs'. Actually, the decision has nothing to do with the pros and cons – it has to do with what is medically right for you. So listening to your surgeon is very important. Once you choose your surgeon, you have to trust him (a point I will return to because I think it is important). Otherwise, you will be going around in circles, and that is very exhausting.

My surgeon also did not tell me much about the sort of mastectomy that I would be having, which again was frustrating and caused me a lot of anxiety, because naturally, I wanted to know, so that I could mentally prepare myself for it. After a few months, I realised that the reason my surgeon was telling me so little about my future mastectomy was because there are many, many ways to perform a mastectomy, all depending on the individual's cancer and medical needs. Literally many – it all depends on what type of cancer you have, where it is in your body, how big your tumour is, how your skin has healed from radiotherapy (if you have radiotherapy), which is covered later in this chapter.

The factors that go into making this decision are endless. Eventually, I concluded that the most important thing was to get rid of the cancer in my breast and then, only then, when that was done, to start thinking about the reconstruction and the cosmetic side of things.

So I guess what I am trying to say here is that you really do have to have patience and take one step at a time. The thought of losing a breast is initially horrific and it's understandable to want to know exactly what is going to happen and immediately to visualise your outcome – but it is not possible. I truly wish this had been explained to me more clearly, and then I would have avoided so much anxiety.

You have to remember that treatment is a series of steps: assessments, results and *then* decisions based on results.

MASTECTOMY / LUMPECTOMY

When I had my mastectomy, I was given a 'temporary' implant, called an 'extender'. Many people do not need radiotherapy which means they can go ahead and have the full reconstruction at the time of the mastectomy. I had to have radiotherapy a few weeks after my mastectomy, and as you will see in the next chapter, one of the side-effects of radiotherapy is that it can damage your skin and surrounding tissues. Therefore it could damage a newly implanted and reconstructed breast which would cause a host of problems.

So instead, as I have explained, I was given the extender which would stretch my skin and prepare it for a proper reconstruction the following year. It would also give my surgeon time to monitor my skin and see how it was recovering from radiotherapy which would give him an idea of how my body would react to reconstruction. One of the things you don't want is trouble or rejection of your reconstruction.

Just as there are many types of breast cancers, so there are many types of reconstructions.

COLEMAN FAT TRANSFER

Six months after the mastectomy, when it had healed enough, I had a Coleman fat transfer. Minute fat cells are taken from an area, under general anaesthetic where there was 'spare' fat – in my case buttocks and thighs – and implanted into the breast to grow into soft tissue to help replace what has been removed. This is not a form of liposuction – and you are left incredibly bruised around your upper thighs and bottom. Your breast is also left extremely swollen and bruised – but all these things heal over the next few weeks. It's worth the pain, in order to get a good outcome that you'll have to live with forever.

NIPPLE

There are many ways to re-create the nipple. For example you can have a surgical operation where they pinch up the skin to make it look like a nipple, and then they tattoo the areola around it. Or you can do what is known as a 'nipple share' where some of your nipple is removed from your good breast and used to make the nipple on your new breast. There are many ways to go about this.

To me a new nipple wasn't important at this stage. I felt I had had so much surgery that I decided to wait to have it done. And needless to say, I have done nothing about it yet. But I do have a wonderful prosthetic nipple that I slip on if I am wearing something sheer, so that both sides match! You can buy them in all shapes and sizes. I have found these invaluable (see plate).

LIVER OPERATION

A few months after my mastectomy and a few weeks after my radiotherapy (which I cover in the next chapter) had finished, I had an operation on my liver, designed to destroy tumours which had spread using a procedure called RFA – Radio Frequency Ablation.

A special extremely hot rod was inserted through the side of my body and the tumours were all blasted away. I had to stay only one or two nights in hospital (I can't remember exactly how long), and I was doing a backward dive (see plate) 10 days later! This really was a spontaneous and defining moment for me, cleverly caught on camera by my daughter.

From diagnosis through to the end of my non-surgical treatment it was only 11 months and it was 18 months to complete all the surgeries (bar the nipple and areola reconstruction).

My oncologist is hoping that the cancer in my bone has been contained by the chemotherapy – so no more operations there, thank goodness. I couldn't believe that I had had so much treatment and surgeries in such a short space of time.

THINGS THAT CAN GO WRONG

After everything that my body had been through over 18 months, I think I fared pretty well, but of course things don't always go to plan. Below I discuss infection risks, cording, capsular contracture, lymphoedema and seromas.

It does pay to be vigilant about your healing process and to check for anything that doesn't seem quite normal. Don't be afraid to ask or go back and see your surgeon, or ring the breast care nurses.

SEROMA

A seroma is a build-up of clear fluids in a place where tissue has been removed by surgery. Seromas look like giant blisters – and when I say giant, I mean giant, like the size of a tangerine.

Seromas can appear seven to ten days after surgery. Most seromas are reabsorbed back into your body after about a month. But sometimes you have to get them drained back in the hospital.

I got a seroma under my armpit where they had taken away the sentinel lymph nodes after my triple lumpectomy. I had never heard of a seroma before and was quite shocked and scared. It was extremely painful and it was decided that it should be drained, rather than be naturally absorbed back into the system. The doctors had wanted to see if it would be naturally absorbed back into the body because draining a seroma carries quite a risk of infection and also doesn't allow the remaining lymph nodes 'learn' to drain!

The seroma happened because the fluids in my body had not adapted to finding the lymph nodes behind the ones that were removed, and the fluid was piling up where the removed ones used to be (see plate).

You must keep an eye on your seroma if you have one, making sure there are no signs of infection, such as redness, warmth or tenderness.

INFECTION

Your surgeon will tell you that there is always a risk of infection with surgery. I would highly recommend insisting on a course of antibiotics after surgery. For no apparent reason (as I had a pretty strong immune level and was doing all the right things) I had a nasty infection after my breast reconstruction and I had to go back into hospital

10 days after, for a week, and be on a drip of antibiotics.

It was very disappointing because I really thought I had seen the last of hospitals for a while. I had planned a lovely Easter for my husband and the children, and ended up in hospital for the whole period. I then had to take very strong antibiotics for six weeks after. If I had taken a short course of strong antibiotics straight after the operation, this probably would not have happened.

CAPSULAR CONTRACTURE

Your surgeon will have informed you that this is a possible risk.

After having the breast implant, your body creates a capsule of fibrous scar tissue around the implant as part of the healing process. This is a natural reaction that occurs when any foreign object is surgically implanted into the body.

Over time, the scar tissue will begin to shrink. This shrinkage is known as capsular contraction. The rate and extent at which the shrinkage occurs varies from person to person. In some people, the capsule can tighten and squeeze the implant, making the breast feel hard. You may also experience pain and discomfort. It may affect the appearance of your new breast.

There is no rhyme or reason as to who experiences this. But if it happens, you may need a further adjustment of the implants. There are several ways to do this, and your surgeon will recommend to you the best way to proceed.

LYMPHOEDEMA

Lymphoedema refers to swelling that generally occurs in your arm.

It is caused by a blockage in your lymphatic system, an important part of your immune and circulatory systems. The blockage prevents lymphatic fluid from draining well, and as the fluid builds up, the swelling continues. Lymphoedema is most commonly caused by the removal of or damage to your lymph nodes as a part of surgery or treatment, such as radiotherapy.

Lymphoedema can occur within a few days, months, or years after surgery. A small amount of swelling is normal for the first four to six weeks after surgery. There is no cure for lymphoedema, but it can be controlled.

How to prevent or control lymphoedema:

- Maintain good nutrition
- Exercise regularly
- Avoid infections
- Avoid heavy lifting with the part of your body that has had the surgery
- Lymphatic drainage massage

- Self lymphatic drainage (I always stroke and lightly massage my right arm; it's a sort of automatic reaction and I'm sure it helps – very light skin brushing does too)
- Avoid extreme temperature changes (saunas, jacuzzis and very hot baths, etc.)
- Compression garments for sport

CORDING

Cording can happen straight after surgery or even months later. It's an uncomfortable feeling as if a tight cord is running from your armpit, down the inner arm and often to the palm of your hand, and is thought to be caused by hardened lymph vessels. Stretching the cord can be very helpful, as is physiotherapy.

EXERCISES AFTER SURGERY

The day after both of my breast surgeries, a physiotherapist appeared in my room and started me on exercises specifically to help regain movement in my arm and shoulders. It was all part of the aftercare connected to my surgery.

It is very important to do these exercises, as not only will it have a positive impact on your well-being but it will help to:

- alleviate symptoms of cording
- increase your range of movement
- encourage the lymphatic system to work more efficiently, thereby reducing the risk of cording
- reduce the possibilities of long-term stiffness and incorrect posture

Your physiotherapist will tell you how long you should do these exercises for. If you're unsure, talk to your breast nurse. They are not difficult to do; however, they may feel uncomfortable to begin with. But you will be amazed at what you can achieve within a few days.

HOSPITAL KIT LIST FOR SURGERY

As with chemo it is very important to make sure you are as comfortable as possible in hospital, so here is a kit list which will help remind you of what to take:

- Slippers and bed socks
- Dressing gown
- Several pairs of loose-fitting PJs with buttons down the front – for easy access for the cannula
- Your favourite shawl, poncho or cardy
- If you are a bit fussy about your pillow – bring one in!

- Blanket from home
- Pillow sprays (gets rid of that hospital laundry smell)
- Chargers
- iPads, laptops, books and magazines

And most importantly, do not have too many visitors or phone calls. Use this time in hospital to get as much rest as possible.

7
Radiotherapy

Radiotherapy uses high levels of radiation to kill cancer cells or keep them from growing and dividing – while minimising damage to healthy cells. It is given to reduce your risk of local recurrence of the cancer for which you are being treated. The treatments generally start several weeks after the surgery so the area has had some time to heal. If your doctor recommends chemotherapy along with radiotherapy, this might be given before you start radiotherapy.

Once radiotherapy treatments start, you can expect to receive small daily doses of radiation five days a week over a period of three to six weeks.

BEFORE TREATMENT STARTS

You will be asked to go to the radiotherapy unit before your sessions of radiotherapy begin. You will have to lie down on a machine where radiographers will spend a bit of time getting you in the correct position and taking measurements for your future treatment. This involves lining up the lasers that will give you your treatment. They will tattoo a few tiny pin pricked size marks on your body. It does not hurt. (This outlines the treatment area of your body and lasers are used to line this up – a kind of 'join the dots' thing.) It is almost like they are creating a master map of you so that when you go into your daily radiotherapy sessions, they will be able to get you into the perfect position, in the quickest possible time. Radiotherapy is totally personalized – so the amount and location is prescribed only for you.

I remember this setting up process was quite challenging for me, as I had to lie with my arms up for quite a long time, and since I had just had surgery a few weeks before in my armpit and a triple lumpectomy, followed by a mastectomy and a seroma (which you now know all about), it was quite difficult and tiring but was quite a complicated case with a large area to target. I found it very helpful to deal with these sessions by going into a semi-meditative state.

RADIOTHERAPY SESSIONS

It is very, very cold in the radiotherapy treatment rooms. Again, this is necessary in order to keep these incredible machines cool. Bring in a scarf, woolly socks and a hat. You are normally allowed to wear these, yet nobody tells you this. It makes such a difference.

You will be given a changing room to change into a robe. The radiographer will escort you into the treatment room, help you on to the treatment table and help place you in the correct treatment position. Once the radiographer is sure you are positioned correctly, he or she will leave the room and start the radiation treatment. You will not feel anything! The actual treatment itself only takes a few minutes.

It is the setting up and getting you in position that takes the time. This part is easy for some people and not so for others. It depends where exactly you are being radiated and how intense the treatment is. The nurses always found it incredibly difficult to get me in the correct position, so my radiotherapy sessions took a lot longer, and remaining utterly still in a physically stressful and painful position was extremely testing at times. Sometimes we had to start over which was very depressing.

You will be under constant observation during the treatment. Cameras and an intercom are in the treatment room, so the radiographer can always see and hear you. If you should have a problem, you can let the radiographer know. It is very important that you remain still and relaxed during treatment. Going into my meditative trance really did help enormously.

The radiographer will be in and out of the room to reposition the machine and change your position. The treatment machine will not touch you and, as I said, you will feel nothing during the treatment.

In order to confirm that you are in the right position, the radiographer will take a 'port film', or X-ray, on the first day of treatment and approximately every week thereafter. Port films verify that you are being accurately positioned during your treatments. Port films do not provide diagnostic information, so radiographers cannot learn about your progress from these films. However, port films are important to help the radiographers maintain precision in your treatment (see plate).

SIDE-EFFECTS

EXTREME FATIGUE

I have covered fatigue earlier. My fatigue was extreme, partly, I am sure, because it was the last thing we did in the first year of my treatment. I had already had the chemotherapy and several operations on my breast. By the time radiotherapy came around I had already had several general anaesthetics in a short space of time. By this point I was dead beat!

Personally, I hated radiotherapy, probably even more than the chemo. I found the whole thing claustrophobic and I felt I had absolutely no privacy whilst the nurses were constantly measuring, checking and moving my breast flesh around like bits of meat with their ice cold hands. I know they had to do it and they were simply wonderful – it was just a situation that could not be avoided, but by the time I was getting into my 20th day, the daily journey into my clinic, going through the procedure and getting home again I was simply beyond exhaustion.

Having said all this, many people do not have such bad side-effects. Fatigue may also come at different times from radiotherapy; sometimes it gets even worse after you have finished the course.

To minimise fatigue while you are receiving radiation treatment:

- Be sure to get enough rest
- Eat a well-balanced, nutritious diet
- Pace your activities and plan frequent rest periods
- Carry out small amounts of exercise
- Let other people take you to and from the sessions

SKIN PROBLEMS

In the area exposed to radiation, your skin may become red, swollen, itchy, warm and sensitive – as if you have nasty sunburn. It may peel or become moist and tender. Depending on the dose of radiation you receive, you may notice a loss of hair (yay! the armpit!) or decreased perspiration within the treated area – again, yay!

These skin reactions are common and temporary. They will subside gradually within four to six weeks of completing treatment. Long-term side-effects, which can last up to a year or longer after treatment, may include a slight darkening of the skin, enlarged pores in the treated area, increased or decreased sensitivity of the skin; weaker skin. The skin on your treated side may never look the same as the skin on your untreated side.

HOW TO CARE FOR THE AREA THAT IS BEING TREATED:

- Gently cleanse the treated area using lukewarm water. I used to put moisturiser on first to act as a barrier cream and then get in the bath or shower. Do not submerge treated area in the bath. And if you are showering, just let the water trickle over it as little as possible. The moisturiser would do the job of cleansing rather than soap.

The bath water could only come waist high but it was better than nothing

- Don't rub your skin. Pat your skin dry with a soft towel or use a hairdryer on a cool setting
- Don't scratch or rub the treated area
- Moisturise your skin constantly (I did it about three or four times a day). Only use the ones that your clinic gives or authorises you to use. If you are having any problems at all, you must report them and they may find a different cream for you. The reason you must only use the prescribed cream is because it must not have aluminum or other chemicals in it as this will interfere with the radiotherapy. There were some other creams that I obtained which were more expensive, aluminium-free and felt more comfortable to use. I showed them to the nurses and they were happy for me to use them
- Don't apply cosmetics, shaving lotions, perfumes or deodorants on the treated area
- Use only an electric razor if you need to shave the treated area
- Don't wear tight-fitting clothing or clothes made from fabrics that might irritate your skin for any reason. Instead choose clothes made from soft natural fibres, such as cotton

- Don't apply plasters or bandages to the treated area
- Don't expose the treated area to extreme heat or cold – i.e. hot water bottles or ice packs
- Make sure your baths are not too hot. I found this very difficult as I was always freezing after treatments and longed for boiling hot long baths!
- Keep the treated area out of direct sunlight and always wear a very high factor sunblock – even after your course of treatment has finished

8
Nutrition, Exercise & Alternative Therapies

Let thy food be thy medicine

Hippocrates came up with so many brilliant quotes, and this is one that might be a helpful to bear in mind as you progress through your treatment – and life!

DIET AND NATURAL PREVENTION

Good nutrition is an essential part of recovering from the side-effects of all your treatments for cancer, short-term and long-term. Eating well will help with your energy levels, and help your body to heal and fight infection. Most importantly, good nutrition can give you a sense of well-being. Since eating when you don't feel well can be difficult, a nutritionist can help you find ways to get the nutrients you need during your treatment, even if you are finding it difficult to eat. Make sure you research your nutritionist well. Go by recommendations, and very importantly go to a nutritionist who has a ton of experience in looking after cancer patients.

WILL MY ONCOLOGIST TELL ME ABOUT NUTRITION?

The answer is probably not. He may say, 'Eat well and make sure your diet is healthy.' You can't really expect him to go into the subject of nutrition at great length as his job is life-saving oncology, providing you with gold standard treatment, and not nutrition.

Many hospitals have Cancer Centres within them where dieticians can recommend how and what to eat during treatment and there are booklets covering this, available in hospitals and from cancer charities.

GETTING STARTED

In order for your eating blueprint to be effective, you must first stop doing that which is promoting cancer growth (or poor health in general), and *then* all the other preventive strategies have the chance to really have an impact. So, rather than adding certain foods, you'll want to eliminate the most dangerous culprits first. The most important thing is what you do or do not put in your mouth. You can have huge influence on your health by the foods you consume and the foods that you avoid.

Another important factor in learning to eat healthily is to avoid food with labels! The idea of healthy eating is not to 'read labels' as we are so often advised. If food has all these labels on it, including 'low fat', it means it is full of chemicals and massively processed. So stay away.

There are two important facts to bear in mind when making food choices:

- Cancer cells have an extreme acid pH and are oxygen depleted
- Healthy cells have a slightly alkaline pH and a high oxygen content

AN ALKALINE DIET

This is why I want to focus on an alkaline diet. It is the opposite of an acidic diet and the crux of what I have learnt is that an acidic diet causes inflammation which is the cause of many life threatening diseases, such as cancer.

A highly alkaline diet can alleviate, combat and help prevent many diseases, including autism, arthritis, diabetes and depression. There is overwhelming evidence now, endorsed by many cancer organisations, that diet, exercise and weight control can increase survival and help prevent a cancer returning.

An alkaline diet will oxygenate your body tissues instead of acidifying them. It will feed your body with the vitamins, minerals and nutrients required.

Although the body includes a number of organ systems that are equipped at neutralising and eliminating excess acid, there is a limit to how much acid even a healthy body can cope with effectively. The body is capable of maintaining an acid-alkaline balance provided that the organs are functioning properly, that a well-balanced alkaline diet is being consumed, and that other acid-producing factors are avoided. In short, your body pH affects everything

The alkaline diet greatly reduces the acid in the body, helping to reduce the strain on the body's acid-detoxification systems, such as the kidneys. When body pH drops below 6.4, enzymes are deactivated and digestion does not work properly. Acid decreases energy production in the cells, the ability of the body to repair damaged cells, and its ability to detoxify. You can buy little kits that test the pH of your body so you can see how alkaline you are managing to get yourself.

The benefits of an alkaline diet:

- It does wonders for the digestion and reduces bloatedness
- It improves skin tone
- It promotes better memory, focus and concentration, as blood sugar levels are stabilised

- It promotes better mood as many of the grains satisfy the serotonin receptor sites in the gut, which in turn help to elevate mood
- It produces greatly improved energy levels, as many of the most alkaline foods are slow-release carbohydrates and vegetarian proteins, which help to keep blood sugar balanced more evenly
- It reduces cravings for sugar, alcohol, coffee and other stimulants

Before you get too alarmed, I must stress that it is virtually impossible to follow an alkaline diet (which includes no sugar) 100 per cent. It is a question of common sense, balance and awareness. Follow it as much as you can – try and keep to the 80/20 rule. There will be times when you will break your own rules, but remember: you are only human! I have certainly broken my own rules from time to time, and I don't think I would be able to have continued my diet long term if I *hadn't* broken the rules.

When I was first diagnosed, I followed the diet referred to below more or less 100 per cent and lost two stone. Now I am following it 80/20 and I have put on a bit of weight (which was needed) and feel very happy where I am now.

Going into great detail about what all the right foods to eat would be a book in itself, so here I am listing a few foods to give you an idea of the good ones. I am just giving you pointers, leaving it up you to take it from here. There are many really useful books, and websites on alkalining foods which offer lots of delicious recipes.

VERY ALKALINING FOODS
(EAT IN ABUNDANCE)

- **Beverages** – Green Tea, Vegetable Juice
- **Fruits** – Apples, Avocado, Blackberries, Blueberries, Cantaloupe Melon, Cherries, Grapes, Guava, Lemons, Papaya, Peaches, Pineapple, Plums, Raspberries, Strawberries
- **Herbs & Spices** – Coriander, Garlic, Ginger, Horseradish, Parsley, Turmeric
- **Legumes** – Aduki Beans, Black Beans, Chick Peas, Fava Beans, Green Beans, Green Peas, Lentils, Lima Beans, Mung Beans, Pinto Beans, Red Beans, White Beans
- **Oils & Fats** – Coconut Oil, Extra Virgin Olive Oil, Flaxseed Oil
- **Sea Vegetables** – Agar, Kelp, Wakame
- **Vegetables** – Artichoke, Asparagus, Brussels Sprouts, Beet Greens, Broccoli, Cabbage, Carrot, Cauliflower, Celery, Chard, Cucumber, Endive, Kale, Mushrooms, Radishes, Radicchio, Red Peppers, Rocket, Salad Leaves, Shallots, Spinach , Turnip Greens, Watercress

Most fruits do contain sugar, so it is important to eat proportionately more vegetables than fruit.

NEUTRAL ALKALINING FOODS
(THESE ARE NOT ACIDIC, BUT THEY ARE NOT PARTICULARLY ALKALINING – SO THEY ARE PERFECTLY FINE TO EAT)

- **Dairy & Eggs** – Eggs, Cottage Cheese
- **Grains** – Barley, Buckwheat, Oats, Quinoa, Brown Rice, Spelt, Wild Rice
- **Fruits** – Coconut, Cranberries, Gooseberries, Grapefruit, Kiwi, Mango, Peaches, Pomegranate, Rhubarb, Tangerine, Watermelon
- **Herbs & Spices** – All herbs and spices not mentioned in the section above
- **Nuts & Seeds** – Almonds, Brazil, Cashew, Chestnuts, Macadamia, Pecans, Pistachios, Poppy Seeds, Pumpkin Seeds, Sesame Seeds, Sunflower Seeds, Walnuts
- **Oils & Fats** – Almond Oil, Canola Oil, Sesame Oil
- **Poultry** – Chicken, Turkey, Duck, Goose, Pheasant & Quail
- **Seafood** – Cod, Crayfish, Halibut, Mackerel, Perch, Salmon, Sea Bass, Snapper, Squid, Whitefish

ACIDIC FOODS
(TRY AND AVOID)

These foods can cause acidosis, which is when the body tissue becomes too acidic, and lacks the proper amount of oxygen to keep it healthy. Your body's immune system ends up inflamed and compromised.

RED MEAT – BEEF, PORK, LAMB AND VENISON

Not only is red meat highly acidic, many of the animals that produce this meat are given antibiotics, growth hormones and other veterinary drugs that get stored in their tissues. Additionally, cooking the meat over high heat has a carcinogenic effect. So keep your BBQs to a minimum!

If from time to time, as a major treat, you do have some red meat then you should only entertain the idea of organically-raised, grass-fed meat. (White meat, such as turkey or chicken is not acidic and is fine to eat in small amounts – but again, make sure it is organic.)

SUGAR (THIS INCLUDES ALL FORMS, INCLUDING FRUCTOSE AND GRAINS OTHER THAN WHOLE GRAINS)

Sugar feeds all diseases, and cancer loves it. It is truly the devil. It promotes inflammation and oxygen free radicals. Those are the two main processes that underlie many chronic disorders, including cancers. It fuels the growth of breast cancers, because glucose is cancer's favourite food.

Here is an extraordinary tale: during the 18 months preceding diagnosis, I was feeling very unwell, as I mentioned early – always shattered, bloated and puffy. I formed a sugar addiction. I literally would feel this terrible urge to have sugar and I would attack anything sugary with ferocity. Looking back, that was the cancer craving the sugar to grow – and I was feeding it. How little I knew then!

FATS

Bad fats in the diet are a major contributor to ill health and cancer. On the list of fats to eliminate are: animal fats; trans fats; and partially hydro-genated or hydrogenated fats.

Do not confuse these fats with healthy fats, such as those found in nuts, which are of particular importance for cancer prevention. Omega-3, for example (found in flax seeds, walnuts, sardines, salmon, soybeans, tofu, shrimp, sprouts, cauliflower and winter squash), slows down tumour growth in oestrogen-sensitive cancers such as breast, prostate and colon cancers.

CHEMICALS THAT MIMIC OESTROGEN (XENOESTROGENS)

Avoid canned food and linings of food containers that contain plastic. We have all been warned for a long time about the chemicals that leak out of plastic mineral water bottles when left in the sun (i.e. your car).

DAIRY

It is cow's dairy that you want to avoid, which includes milk, cheese, yoghurts and so on. Cow's milk contains a growth hormone that makes cells grow and divide rapidly. I recently discovered how delicious unsweetened almond milk is – and most supermarkets stock it! Cheese is also highly acidic – keep this to a minimum.

PROCESSED FOODS

Long before I was diagnosed with cancer I started ranting on and on about processed foods. I *loathe* processed foods.

Processed foods are foods that have been changed from their natural state – convenience snack foods, like crisps, and ready meals. If they have a label of ingredients on they are normally processed.

There are many harmful and negative facts about processed food, which include the following: they are highly addictive; they cause chronic inflammation; they ruin digestion; they often contain pesticides and genetically modified ingredients.

Actually, processed foods are not really foods at all – which is quite a scary thing to contemplate. They are man-made. Somebody once said to me, 'Think of it as wearing a natural cotton jumper compared to a nylon one. The nylon one is much less comfortable and does not let your body breathe.' The same with processed foods; they're simply not natural.

Have you noticed how homemade bread grows mould a lot quicker than processed white sliced supermarket bread? Have you noticed how organic salads don't last as long as vacuum packed salads? Basically processed foods last a lot longer than non-processed foods because they have been tampered with, and altered with chemicals and preservatives.

Most of the flavour and colour of processed foods does not come from the natural food but a synthetically produced chemical that replicates the taste and flavor. What a thought! What toll do you think this is taking on our bodies when we try to digest this? Real foods will actually grow mould or rot whereas processed foods will not really change very much in appearance.

One last thing about processed foods: people often say they are cheaper. This is not true. I think people get confused between 'cheapness' and 'convenience'. Cooking from scratch is definitely less expensive and is not too inconvenient if you organise yourself well.

To summarise, try to avoid all processed foods, including:

- processed breakfast cereals (which are low in nutrients and high in sugar and salt)
- commercially produced biscuits, cakes and breads (which are high in yeast, white flour, salt, sugar and additives – all acid-forming components)
- fizzy drinks
- alcohol
- coffee
- chocolate (especially milk chocolate, which is high in sugar and dairy solids)
- red meat, including beef, pork, lamb and venison
- cheese

GENERAL TIPS FOR EVERYONE

These lists above are not exhaustive. Use common sense – and give yourself a few breaks. Mine was to have semi-skimmed milk in my tea and also marmite and a scrape of butter on my toast every other morning. I had granola and almond milk on the other mornings, and sometimes scrambled egg.

I got a bread maker and substituted agave syrup for sugar, and olive oil for butter, and eliminated the salt. Use spelt instead of flour – much better for you. A bread maker is so easy to use.

Eat wholewheat pasta and grains, etc., and eat organic if possible but don't beat yourself up over it. I also buy a lot of my fruit and veg from my greengrocer. A lot of it is not organic but it is local. There are many benefits to buying locally – fewer travel miles so less loss of vital nutrients, for example. Plus, the produce has often come from small farms so has not been so intensively farmed.

SUPPLEMENTS

As mentioned before, I am not a qualified nutritionist, but I have done a lot of research, as you can imagine, and since my diagnosis I have been having regular blood tests, as you have to if you are undergoing chemotherapy. The results are very interesting and I put a lot of the good results down to taking the appropriate supplements.

Blood tests show whether the different compounds of your blood are working properly and within a normal range. For example, sodium, potassium, urea, glucose and cholesterol.

Here are just some of the other things they will check in regular blood tests (there are, of course, many more):

- Haemoglobin, which carries oxygen around the body
- WBC (white blood cells), which fight infection
- Lymphocytes – another type of white blood cell which aids the immune system
- Platlets, which help the blood to clot
- Tumour markers, which *can* be elevated when you have cancer (mine were not!) – there are, in fact, many different types of tumour markers corresponding to the many different types of cancer, and your oncologist knows which ones to look out for
- eGFR (Estimated Glomerular Filtration Rate), which is checked to make sure that the kidneys are working properly and have not been impaired by the medication/treatment

It is extraordinary how not only have my bloods stayed at the same healthy level (since before chemotherapy), but they have actually improved since diagnosis. I am convinced that this is linked to my diet and the supplements that I have been taking.

It is hard to believe that, since starting chemo in November 2011, I have not had a single cold, cough, flu, or stomach bug – despite being surrounded by them during the last few winters.

I do take quite a lot of supplements, but the ones that I consider the top, and to be taken regardless, are as follows.

VITAMIN D3

There's overwhelming evidence that lack of Vitamin D plays a crucial role in cancer development. The evidences shows that you can decrease your chances of developing cancer by half simply by optimising your vitamin D levels with sun exposure.But research also shows that most of the time we do not get enough, so supplements will make up for it. But it has to be a proper amount which should be determined by your nutritionist. I have watched my Vitamin D levels increase dramatically since I started taking the supplement, and they have been and continue to be at a good stable level.

MELATONIN

Melatonin is not only the sleep hormone, but it decreases the amount of oestrogen the body produces, helping to regulate estrogen metabolism. It also acts as an antioxidant to protect DNA against damage during treatments and it boosts the immune system.

ASPIRIN

Recent research appears to show that taking small doses of aspirin not only significantly slows the growth of cancer cells and shrinks tumours, but also stops tumour cells spreading to new sites. But taking asprin is not without risk; for instance, daily aspirin use can increase the risk of gastrointestinal bleeding. So you must always check with your GP or nutritionist and only take a 'baby' aspirin.

BIOCURCUMIN (TUMERIC)

Turmeric is a natural anti-inflammatory; it inhibits the growth of new blood vessels in tumours and it is a powerful antioxidant. It also supports healthy joint function, anti-aging and memory function. It helps improve digestion, keeps cholesterol levels down and promotes healthy blood and liver function. It has been used in India and Sri Lanka for thousands of years.

FISH OIL

Fish oil contains the Omega-3 fatty acids EPA and DHA. These fatty acids are known to reduce inflammation, pain and swelling, as well as having a host of other potential benefits, such as preventing heart disease, macular degeneration and clinical depression. Our bodies do not produce Omega-3 fatty acids and cannot make Omega-3 fatty acids from Omega-6 fatty acids which are common in our diets, which is why it is important to take it as a supplement.

One side-effect of chemotherapy – dry eyes and skin irritation – can also be helped by taking fish oil.

BUYING THE RIGHT SUPPLEMENTS

It is very important that you buy the right type of supplement. I would not advise buying these from your local pharmacy as you have no idea what strength you should be taking. That is why it is very important to see a nutritionist who will be able to recommend the best sources and give you the correct dose. I hear so many people say, 'Oh, I take fish oil,' or, 'My multivitamin tablet contains Vitamin D,' and when I ask them how much, they have no idea. Normally, when I look at their container, the tablet contains minuscule amounts and therefore is not making any difference.

HYDRATION

Hydration is also very important and many alkaline foods are packed with vitamin- and mineral-laden water, which is more easily absorbed than plain bottled or tap water. This allows you to hydrate the body from food and not just from drinking water. As lemon is, surprisingly, one of the most alkaline forming things you can consume, I always have a glass of water with lemon in it on the go all day. I make a special lemon and fresh mint water which I consume in huge quantities.

SLEEP

I understand fully that when you are going through treatment, sleep can be an issue and the medications that are taken can interfere with sleep. But try and get as much sleep and rest as you can.

EMOTIONAL WELL-BEING

Anxiety, stress and worry manifest when the body releases adrenalin which raises the heart rate in order to pump blood to the muscles. Messages are being sent through the neural pathways to those muscles to tense up and get ready for action. Your breathing changes from the stomach to shallow breathing from the chest (which is not proper breathing).

According to psychiatrists, the human body is conditioned to deal and cope with six weeks to three months of stress (depending on the person) before that stress actually begins to manifest itself physically. These symptoms include anxiety, low mood, wanting to hide under the duvet, insomnia, gastric problems, stomach aches, loss of bladder control, loss of or increased appetite, plus psychosomatic symptoms such as eczema, palpitations, headaches, excessive thirst, sweating through the hands/head.

This is the body reacting to stress. Your cortisol levels are raised, and your body is in a way preparing for battle – tensing up. That's why when you are stressed your muscles ache so much and you feel in dire need of a massage. If these physical symptoms and feelings go on for longer than the few weeks I mentioned, then it is very important that you make profound adjustments to the way you are coping.

WAYS OF COUNTERACTING STRESS

COUNSELLING

It does not mean you need years of therapy, sometimes just a one-off meeting, or perhaps three or four sessions are enough – just so that you can understand what is going on and address your issues. With cancer every area of your life is affected, and you have to accept that your role is now different. And your role differs depending where you are in the disease: pre-cancer, during treatment, and after.

You can go down the counselling route at any time during and after your cancer treatment. It is interesting to know that there are two peaks in referrals to counselling during cancer treatment. These are at diagnosis and at the end of treatment.

EXERCISE

Exercise and fresh air are incredibly important. Good blood circulation is vital – it improves the circulation of immune cells and oxygenates the blood. We know that exercise is a powerful antidote – it actually changes the chemistry in our body, releasing endorphins into the blood. It helps regulate cortisol (that horrible hormone that gets released in stressful situations). It helps reduce elevated insulin levels, which creates the sugar environment that encourages the growth and spread of cancer cells. You see how the great culprit sugar comes up again and again and how it is linked? I don't know how many times to say this but cancer (and a host of other illnesses) and sugar are inextricably linked. And it is only just recently that the world seems to be waking up to this fact. Not a moment too soon.

A brisk walk can really dissipate stress and lift the mood, but sometimes it can be quite hard to take exercise during some of the treatment. When I felt really rotten and weak, I just used to do a few rounds of stretches in my room, to keep my circulation moving. I'd lay down with my legs up the wall to help move my blood around – this is actually a yoga position, believe it or not. Getting friends to take you for small walks or strolls can be enough. You mustn't feel you have to really push yourself – that is not a good idea. The point is, to get out and about in the fresh air, no matter how little, and oxygenate the blood.

BREATHING

A few years before I was diagnosed, I learnt to breathe. That was when I started yoga and mediation. At the time of diagnosis I put this into action. It really does work. Empty your lungs (i.e. breath out) to prepare. Then breathe slowly in for five seconds through your nose, and then breathe out slowly for five seconds. Do this about 10 times and repeat two or three time during the day. You can use this method to relax yourself, anytime and anywhere. I used it a lot in radiotherapy.

My father told me very recently that, when he had to go into hospital for an operation which he was worried about, he remembered me telling him about breathing, and how it had worked so well for him. Such a simple mechanism, he thought.

COMPLEMENTARY THERAPIES

Complementary therapies are often used alongside conventional cancer treatment. They are not used in any way to 'cure' cancer, but to boost physical and emotional health. They can also relieve some of the side effects of the treatments, help you sleep better and reduce stress and anxiety.

MASSAGE

Massage is one of the oldest forms of complementary therapies.

I found massage to be intensely relieving. I would instruct the masseur as to how much pressure I wanted, which actually was quite a lot in my case because my muscles were so tensed up, rock hard. My body ached so much during treatment that, along with yoga and short walks, the massage contributed immensely to my general physical comfort.

Other than the obvious effects of massage (de-stressing, muscles relaxing etc.), it is extremely good for you because it gets your blood flowing around your body, thereby improving your circulation – which we know is really beneficial.

Obviously the masseur must be made aware of where you have had surgery and what condition your health is in and treat you accordingly. But many masseurs (outside the cancer world) will refuse even to touch you if they know you are undergoing chemotherapy. They do not understand chemotherapy (and why should they?); and they do not make any allowances for it. It can be extremely frustrating arriving somewhere to have a massage, only to find that they won't give it to you. So to avoid disappointment you must check that the masseur knows your current health situation and is prepared to treat you.

ACUPUNCTURE

Acupuncture is a Chinese based therapy which has been used for thousands of years. It is based on the belief that an energy, or 'life force', flows through the body in channels called meridians. This life force is known as Qi (pronounced 'chee'). Acupuncturists believe that when Qi cannot flow freely through the body, this can cause illness and that acupuncture can restore the flow of Qi, and so restore health.

Acupuncture involves the insertion, to various depths, of very thin needles through the patient's skin at specific points on the body. It is not known how acupuncture works scientifically. However, it is acknowledged to have many therapeutic benefits, including pain relief and alleviation from nausea caused by chemotherapy. I did not use acupuncture because my whole treatment was and still is, based around needles – and I hate needles!

REFLEXOLOGY

Reflexology is related to acupuncture. It involves applying pressure to the feet, with specific thumb, finger, and hand techniques. It is based on what reflexologists claim to be a system of zones and reflex areas that they say reflect an image of the body on the feet and hands, with the supposition that such work effects a physical change to the body.

I have always loved reflexology. I am very lucky that the place where I have my cancer treatment has a reflexologist who comes around when you are having treatment and administers it. I battle with insominia but I find this a deeply relaxing treatment and often fall asleep – much to the amazement of everybody! Some or all of these therapies are often offered as part of your care in hospital wards, community health services and various cancer charities.

YOGA

One of my friends, who is a yoga teacher, used to come round and give me very mild yoga lessons. I cannot stress enough how beneficial I found this – from the exercise point of view and spiritually. It is a fantastic way to stay calm and centred; to teach yourself to truly relax and focus and be in the moment. All of these things, I am convinced, have helped me no end. I used to practise yoga before my diagnosis and I still do.

Just by doing a few easy yoga poses in your bedroom; for example, you will be getting your circulation going, stretching and toning your muscles. It gives you the effect of having a massage – but for free!

MEDITATION AND MINDFULNESS

It's not just what you put in your mouth that is important, but also what you put in your mind.

You must have faith in your treatment, fill your heart with love, allow yourself to be loved and get rid of fear. Fear has a negative impact on your well-being.

As with yoga, I found, and still find, meditation invaluable. You can meditate almost anywhere – at actual classes or at your desk, in your bedroom, in the bath, on the bus, and so forth. You can adapt it to suit you – that's the beauty of it.

If you have not meditated before, here is a 'quick guide' to meditation, composed by a dear friend of mine when she took notes when we went on a meditation day together

Meditation technique in four steps:

1. RELAX INTO YOUR POSTURE – becoming present (mindful), with attention turned up
2. TUNE INTO STILLNESS – connect to awareness. (Stillness *is* awareness – witness the mind, but don't react to it. A sense of

stillness is the opposite of feeling scattered. Find equanimity.)

3. SETTLE LIKE WATER – leave everything as it is, stilling the heart and coming to a place of peace. Like water, leave it to settle. Neither accept nor reject what arises – you can only do this when the mirror (the surface of the lake) is undisturbed. The moment we react, the mind cannot see clearly what it is (like ripples on the surface of the water). When the mind is still, we can see clearly.

4. PLACE ATTENTION IN ONE PLACE = concentration.

When meditating, thoughts arise – should we investigate them? Let them go. Be with uncomfortable feelings – they pass – if we can allow ourselves to let them go. Life is about the rough and the smooth, ups and downs.

The practice is to find the capacity to be with things we find hard to be with. Stability within instability. This takes time, effort and courage. Equanimity is leaving things as they are – it is our reaction to 'stuff' that disturbs us. Be with what it is.

Keep reminding yourself, every challenge is an opportunity to evolve.

9
Recovery

You are probably at your most exhausted and rundown post-treatment and wondering, 'What next?' You will be trying to do more physical and mental things and getting back to normal with your everyday life, which is immensely tiring.

It takes a long time to get over the effects of chemotherapy and radiotherapy, and sometimes it is very difficult for the people around you to appreciate this. So this is the time to really try to look after number one! And by doing this, you are actually helping all those around you who depend on you too. And just say 'no' to things. 'I am not able to do that right now.' Plan your social life around your needs. Leave dinners and other social events early if you are feeling tired. You really have to understand that at this moment you may not be as strong as you would wish to be.

People may treat you as if you are 'better', but in fact this can be the worst time. I found that I couldn't concentrate or focus (effects of the chemotherapy and radiation); my brain was still very fuzzy. I certainly didn't feel capable of driving. All the toxins had built up and I, for one, suddenly felt quite alone. This is a time when you really need empathy and understanding. The best thing to do is make sure that those around you understand this – that you are just beginning to heal.

Having said that, a fellow cancerite rang me recently and said to me, 'I know you are recovering because I hear you are arguing with Carletto again! That's great! That's a really good sign!'

Relationships can change once you enter into the Recovery Stage. During my months of chemo and radiation, I got weaker and weaker, more and more exhausted and I didn't really have a voice. But once I got stronger my 'voice' came back.

You also will change. It's a very common occurrence, but once you've been through the harsh reality of cancer treatment; when you come out the other side, you realise how precious life is and how you will not quietly accept the things that you had previously brushed under the carpet for an easier life. The old you may have trundled on because 'that is what you do', but the new you may not be quite so ready to accept that any more. That is quite normal. In fact it is referred to as 'the new normal'. You will have to get used to the 'new normal' and so will those around you.

People may expect that things will just slot back to how they were before – but don't be surprised if they don't. This can leave you feeling out of sorts and also be an anti-climax. It is a good idea to be prepared for this and to lower any expectations that things will be like the 'old' normal.

Some of the important relationships in your life can change. This can be positive. If there is a bit of turbulence in your relationships with your loved ones, don't panic – things should even themselves out. If it doesn't then perhaps this would be time for some counselling. At the same time, try not to expect too much from your partner. No matter how much she/he is 'with you' on this journey, she/he will never know what it is really like to be in this position.

I found, that at this stage, I actually had time to think about what had happened and the ghastliness of it all. During the previous months I had focused on just getting through the treatment and staying well. I hadn't had the time or even the inclination to analyse what had happened. I found (only momentarily, thank goodness) that this was when the questions came flooding in: Why? Why me? What if I'd insisted on a mammogram a year before? Why didn't my local GP pick it up – I had been feeling unwell for at least two years? Why didn't I know or take on board that my long-deceased grandmother and aunt had had breast cancer? Why had I had the test for ovarian cancer and not looked into breast cancer? How long am I going to live? Am I going to be a statistic?

The questions are endless. There is no real an-swer – it is what it is. And I feel the best way forward at this juncture is to accept what has happened and continue to put all my energies into staying well and recovering. You must have no room in your life for bitterness and anger. Instead you thank God for every beautiful day you have.

Conclusion

So, what *has* cancer taught me?

According to Kalil Kibran, 'You are good when you walk to your goal firmly and with bold steps.' Happiness is made up of small things in a day – little rituals which tell you to stop, look and listen to your own breathing. This is what my illness has taught me. My body is a magical thing, with a life of its own, part of the great universe and the mystery of life. I have learned to live with cancer, to harness it. Being so ill has taught me the humility to accept the love that so many people have poured around me and my precious family.

There is a grace about receiving this love and letting go of your independence while you heal yourself. Allowing other people to comfort me when they see someone they love in such a dark place, has made me a better, more loving human being.

I have re-connected with the awesome beauty and power of nature. I have seen the wonder of the hundreds of remarkable people who have lovingly enfolded me in their care, their skills, their brains – and their being there for me with selfless devotion has brought me gently to a state of contentment and real happiness I have never known before.

Like many other people who have been on this kind of journey I want to share what I have learnt with others who are only just beginning to wonder what lies ahead.

The great sage Seneca said, 'If the anvil is never struck the sparks will never fly.' Around me I see light and love and energy and above all, fear has no place in the beauty of my life.

This is what I have learnt from cancer.

Further Information

CHARITIES

The wonderful thing about most of the cancer charities is that they 'talk' to and work with each other. So if one particular charity can't fulfil a certain role, they'll call another to see if they can help. It's fantastic to see how they work together with such an unfailing team spirit.

Breast Cancer Breakthrough
www.breakthrough.org.uk
National charity focusing on saving lives through improving early diagnosis, developing new treatments and preventing all types of breast cancer

Breast Cancer Haven
www.thehaven.org.uk
National charity providing emotional, physical and practical support including complementary therapies, counselling, nutritional advice, financial advice and support groups

Cancer Research
www.cancerresearch.org.uk
National charity conducting research into cancer causes and cures. It also provides information on

all types of cancer, treatments, symptoms and preventing cancer

CLIC Sargent
www.clicsargent.org.uk
The UK's leading children's cancer charity providing information, support, practical help, financial assistance and advice

Macmillan Cancer Relief
www.macmillan.org.uk
National charity providing support at all levels for people, families and communities affected with cancer. They provide nurses and other specialist health care professionals guiding patients through the system. They also publish a huge range of booklets on every aspect of the disease and give emotional and practical support including financial help

Maggie's
www.maggiescentres.org
Maggie's has 15 centres (with four in development) nationwide. It provides help from a range of professional people specialising in practical, emotional, and physical support for the patient, family and friends

Marie Curie Cancer Care
www.mariecurie.org.uk

Providing nursing care to give people with all terminal illnesses the choice of dying at home, supported by their families

SPECIALIST WEBSITES

www.acidalkalinediet.net
This website goes into great detail about the benefits of an alkaline diet

www.afmhealth.com (Applied Functional Medicine)
Bob Jacobs, a Naturopath is the driving force behind AFM specialising in promoting immune system function, hormone balance, brain chemistry, metabolism and energy levels

www.chemoheadwear.co.uk
A beautiful range of high quality hats, bandanas and turbans

www.getsomeheadspace.com
A meditation course in the form of an app which leads you through a series of 10-minute meditation practices

www.theartofmeditation.org
Burgs has been teaching meditation in Europe and Asia since 1995, and has hosted over 100 retreats from five days to five months. He offers many meditation courses online too

www.theorganicpharmacy.com
Suppliers of organic health and beauty products

www.trendco.co.uk
A leading supplier of wigs and hairpieces – natural
and synthetic

Acknowledgements

There are many people I need to thank, starting with Naim Attallah of Quartet Books, my publisher – who when I first mentioned the idea of writing my book was so enthusiastic that he gave me the confidence to complete it. He has made this whole project so seamless for me and is a man who turns dreams into reality.

My editor, Elspeth Sinclair, so very subtly skilled and with whom I shared several emotional experiences sitting at her kitchen table going through my book.

My agent, Margaret Hanbury, who whipped it out of my hands and paved the way to publication with incredible efficiency.

And the superb team at Quartet Books, particularly Gavin and Grace. My mother, Vanessa Hannam, who read my book, tactfully critiqued it and quietly in the background steered me in the right direction. She was always there to guide me.

Dr Martin Scurr, my GP, who was there the minute I was diagnosed. He enabled the chain of medical excellence that I have received, and has been a constant godsend to me.

Mr Gerald Gui, my surgeon, whose clinical and surgical excellence has been critical to my recovery and return to good health, through my many operations. He is an artist.

Professor Paul Ellis, my oncologist, at the LOC (Leaders in Oncology Care) in London. The moment I walked into his office for the first time, on that dreadful day when I had been told my cancer had spread, I had a good feeling. Why? His expertise, care and attention, medical brilliance and creative thinking proved a stunning combination.

The unwavering cheerfulness and profession-alism of the staff and nurses at the LOC. And all the nurses at the various hospitals and clinics whose support I received through my unimagina-ble journey, which has helped me to achieve the impossible.

Dr Eva Dubin, founder of the Dubin Breast Center, Mount Sinai Hospital in New York – for all her help and advice.

Henry Dreher, an independent journalist and consultant, who researched on my behalf and gave me extensive advice on the vast range of choices available in conventional treatment, sup-plemental medicine as well as new developing technologies.

The Tumour Vaccine Group, University of Seattle, under which I have enrolled in a groundbreaking and hopefully life-extending trial.

Dr Robert Jacobs, my nutritionist and naturo-path, who has provided me with an invaluable diet and daily regime to help keep my immune system strong. Through him, I have learnt so much about general good health.

My family, especially my three brave children who just 'got on' and still do 'get on' with life in their ebullient way. My father, John Wauchope, and his wife Juliet. Again, my mother Vanessa, my step-father John; my sisters, Ali and Bella, and brother, Andy – for looking after me and being there 24/7.

My dear Angie – the quiet angel. I cannot imagine life without her.

The unswerving loyalty and compassion of my friends; the endless comfort and practical help they have provided and still do. And my new friends; special friendships that I have made along this journey with people I feel as if I've known forever – you know who you are!

Countless remarkable strangers I have come across who have helped me in so many difficult situations.

The teachers and head teachers at my children's schools, who have made it so much easier for me knowing that my children are given pastoral care that is second to none.

Alfred & Judy Taubman – for their introduction to the medical community at the Taubman Institute at the University of Michigan, to which I am eternally grateful.

Sibilla Clark – my mother-in-law, without whom I would not have met many of my medical contacts in the USA.

And lastly, darling Carletto – he should be first on the list, of course, but I want to savour him for last so it is fresh with the reader. It has been a traumatic ride, and still is, for both of us. He has been my rock throughout and must take much of the credit for where I am now. I love you all the way to the moon and back.

Printed in Great Britain
by Amazon